C.J. Rupert Juta

State of Mind, and Homeopathy.

How you think and feel, will govern what you do and who you are.

Disclaimer.

This book is a result of a lot of personal experiences, and also the collection of information from other sources, books, the internet, word of mouth, experiments on the family and friends, and a general interest in Homeopathy and Psychology. Not everything here has been verified by the author, and some of it is purely his own or the opinion of other people. The author is active in sport, life and work, and has seen amazingly good results with Homeopathy, and now uses emotional remedies as a primary treatment for numerous disorders, as did Dr Bach with his Flower Remedies. They are excellent for the mind, emotions and body, and may have a very positive effect on the entire personality.

The suggestions here are mainly to do with acute, or rapidly appearing disorders, and remedies are selected on that basis. Disorders which are chronic, having been there for years, perhaps, may need more in depth repertorisation than this book allows for. However, this book may save you a lot of time searching through other books.

The guidelines which appear here, are not meant as a replacement for a proper Repertory and Materia Medica, but may assist any layperson considerably.

To order additional copies, please contact us.
Booksurge Publishing
www.booksurge.com
orders@booksurge.com

C.J. Rupert Juta

State of Mind, and Homeopathy.

Comprising a Homeopathic Guide to be used for Mental and Emotional strengthening and healing.

C. J. Rupert Juta

2008

The scientist says, "With my self-made rules and word games, I will prove that Homeopathy does not work".

The Homeopath looks at the untold millions of happy people healed by Homeopathy, in numerous different countries, over the centuries, and laughs.

Juta, C.J.Rupert: "Can you Think or are you Programmed?". Booksurge Publishing, USA. 2008.

State of Mind, and Homeopathy. You can change who you are, and how you feel, and what you can accomplish.

MAHATMA GANDHI declared that, "Homeopathy. . . cures a larger percentage of cases than any other method of treatment and is beyond all doubt safer, more economical, and the most complete medical science.

DIGNITARIES WHO HAVE SUPPORTED HOMEOPATHY —IN THE PAST:

Mahatma Gandhi
William James
John D. Rockefeller
Henry Wadsworth Longfellow
Daniel Webster
Harriet Beecher Stowe
Samuel F.B. Morse

IN THE PRESENT:

Queen Elizabeth II, Queen of England
Tina Turner, Singer. Actress
Yehudi Menuhin, Master Violinist
Nicholos Von Hoffman, Syndicated Columnist
William Tiller. Ph.D., Stanford Professor
Pat Riley, Coach of the L.A. Lakers
Lindsay Wagner, Actress
Andrew Weil, M.D., Researcher and Author
OJ Simpson, Football Superstar
Jim Bouton, Ex-Yankee Pitcher
Bob MacAdoo, NBA Rookie-Of-The-Year 1972
Sally Little, Pro Golfer
Kate Schmidt, Two Time Olympic Medallist in The Javelin

C.J. Rupert Juta

For Jeanette and Coen, my parents, and Alison, Ursula, Conrad, Chris and Kumi.

Mark Twain once said, "You may honestly feel grateful that Homeopathy survived the attempts of the allopaths (orthodox physicians) to destroy it." Harper's Magazine, February 1890.

1. Note.

Homeopathy is not a replacement for orthodox medicine, and should be used in conjunction with it, and with other complementary therapies, for optimum life performance. It may assist people to maintain excellent good health, motivation, interest, focus, energy, and good spirits and attitude. Not only can homeopathy help rapid repair of injuries, but it can also calm many of the problems of the mind and emotions, which interfere with happy living.

2. The Calling of the Homeopath.

My calling as a practitioner of the art of homeopathic medicine, is to encourage the Vital Force within all entities, to function as it was designed to do, and to recognise and destroy all morbid influences which threaten its integrity, and lead to disease. I undertake to respect and honour this spirit, wherever it is found, and to help restore the connection between all entities on this planet. I undertake not to accept the limitations posed by words and culture, politics and species, and to make my mind receptive to the greater powers and energies everywhere. To this end I will study continuously, co-operating with the Tao, or natural flow of power, healing each entity with individualized attention and remedies, and teaching these principles to whoever is able to absorb them.
C.J.Rupert Juta

3. The history of this book.

Over the years the author has become increasingly aware that state of mind is the basis for survival, achievement, fame, money, sport awards, peace of mind, fulfilment and much more.
The old adage, "you can if you think you can", has taken on a new dimension. If you think you can, or if the dream is clear enough, then you probably can achieve it. If you think you can't, then you will probably never achieve it. Homeopathy can help you to self-confidence, positive thinking and greater achievements. You may be able to stop vascillating and putting things off, and get into action with Homeopathy. Homeopathy may help you to clear out circular thoughts, pre-occupations, negative pre-conceptions and crippling anxieties.
If the mind is unhealthy, the body tends to become unhealthy, and if the body is unhealthy, the mind tends to be adversely affected. You may be able to help them both function in perfect harmony, by using Homeopathy.
***

Index of information.
***

***

4. List of disorders.
***

It is advisable to consider as many options as possible, when browsing the alphabetical listing..
***

A.
***

Abandoned.
Ability.
Abnormality, obsessed with own strangeness..
Abrasiveness.
Absenteeism to avoid confrontation.
Abstract, unreal fantasies.
Abula (Ebula)..
Affection.
Aggression.
Agoraphobia.
Ailing constantly.
Alienated.
Alone, wants peace and quiet, expects to be cared for.
Alone, fearful.
Aloof.
Ambition, none.
Ambition thwarted, at crossroads.
Amorous frenzy.
Anger, burning deep..
Anger, exhaustion, remorse.
Angry with himself.
Anguish, terrible.
Anti-social.
Anxiety.

Apathy.
Apathy, living death.
Apologetic.
Apprehension, melancholia, doubts, confusion.
Apprehension (see Anxiety).
Apprehension, too much happening at once.
Approval needed all the time.
Arguments in the head.
Arrogance.
Attention, ADHD, ADD.
Attachment to things, excessive.
Aversions.
Awkward.
***

B.
***
Backward, daft, silly.
Begrudges.
Belonging, no sense of.
Bereavement, emotional shock.
Bereavement, grief.
Bewildered.
Bi-polar disorder.
Biting people.
Bitterness, resentment.
Blemish.
Bottled up feelings.
Breakdown constantly feared.
Broken up.
Broodiness.
Brooding.

Bulimia.
Bullying and insensitive.
Burden, believes erroneously.
Burdened, unfairly.
***
C.
***
Calamity expected, no reason.
Camaraderie with others not possible.
Careworn.
Changeability.
Changes personality or character.
Character traits.
Chatting not possible.
Cheerful front.
Cherished surroundings lost.
Childish behaviour.
Claustrophobia with life.
Cleans obsessively.
Clingy, weepy.
Close, too close when speaking.
Closed-minded, dogmatic.
Commanding others.
Complacent, no urgency, just sits.
Complains constantly when ill.
Complaints quashed.
Comprehension so slow, can't understand.
Compulsive.
Concentration (see Attention).
Concerned about others, too much.
Condescending.

Confidence (gone).
Confrontation avoided at all costs.
Confusion.
Confusion about the future is intolerable.
Confusion, shrieks.
Confusion, unreal feeling.
Conscientious, over-conscientious, obstinate.
Consolation, aggravates grief and disappointment.
Consolation constantly sought.
Consolation makes everything worse.
Conspiracy, imagines.
Constricted feeling, squashed.
Contempt.
Contradiction (intolerance to).
Contradictory symptoms.
Contradicts non-stop.
Control, emotional control absent.
Conversation blockage, unable to chat.
Coping, cannot cope anymore.
Cravings.
Crawling round floor.
Creatures creeping in the dark, ghosts.
Closed-minded, dogmatic.
Condescending.
Control, absent mentally.
Conversation blockages.
Crisis, still in shock.
Critical of everything.
Cruel.
Crying does not happen.
***

D.
***

Day-dreaming, instead of working.
Dazed, not with it.
Dead inside, perhaps from grief.
Decisions, too scared to make them.
Defects, certain she has critical defects.
Defiant when given instructions.
Delay impossible, gets frantic.
Delegate, completely unable to.
Delirium, mania, fears of rats.
Delusions (see Winning).
Demands on him excessive.
Dementia.
Depression (see Melancholia).
Depression with fear.
Despair.
Despondent, whining, peevish.
Destructive rage.
Detail, obsessed with.
Determination to succeed.
Devastated.
Devotion to duty not appreciated.
Devotion to loved ones drained out.
Diplomacy absent.
Direction in the passage of life.
Direction, keeps losing it, coming back again.
Disappointment.
Direction, sense of direction fails, lost.
Disappointment (huge).
Disaster, constantly feels disaster is on the way.

Disconsolate, cries for nothing.
Discontented, failing ambitions.
Discontent, permanent feeling of.
Discouraged (see Nervous breakdown).
Disdainful.
Disgruntled person
Disharmony, cannot tolerate.
Disillusioned, cannot tolerate.
Disillusioned, frustrated.
Dislike, of self.
Disobedience to authority.
Dispirited, mental fatigue.
Displeasure and capriciousness at everything.
Disregarded, so angry.
Distracted, unsettled, influenced.
Distraught about welfare of others.
Disturbed mind.
Dogmatic.
Dominance and power.
Dominating position.
Doubts everyone and everything.
Dread, fear, anxiety.
Dread, nervous dread about tomorrow.
Dread of what may happen.
Dreams.
Dreams transformed into reality.
Drive for accomplishment.
Drive gone.
Driven to high standards of work
Duality, two people inside her.
Dull, slow, weak, sad.

Duty, owed to him.
Dying, convinced he is.
Dying, illogically expecting to die shortly.
***
E.
***
Eating compulsion.
Ecstasy, gaiety.
Emotions cast aside for pragmatism.
Emotions (Chinese medicine).
Emptiness of the heart, after loss.
Enlarged objects of vision.
Enmity chronically repressed.
Enraged with the injustice of the system.
Enthusiasm gone.
Envy/hatred.
Escapism, mental, unable to focus on life.
Exams, gradings, trials, terrors.
Example setting.
Excessive behaviour patterns.
Excitement (too much leaves her ill).
Exhilaration, persecution, bliss, untidy.
Exploited people.
Exultation, exaggeration and imagination.
Eye-contact, avoids.
***
F.
***
Façade.
Failure anticipated in everything planned.
Failure, fear of.

Fanatical.
Fate, terrified of possible fate.
Fatigue, incoherence.
Fault-finding obsession.
Fearful of imagined or possible diseases.
Fears (acute, sudden, disrupting).
Fears, acute or sudden.
Fervent, too much.
Fighting, violence, disrupts everyone..
Fixated.
Fixed behaviour patterns.
Fixed in routines and surroundings.
Floating on air.
Flying (fear of).
Follower.
Foreboding.
Fortitude absent.
Fragility, emotional.
Frantic activity and rage.
Fulfilment out of reach.
Futility.
***
G.
***
Gargoyles laughing and shrieking.
Getting going, unable to.
Gloom.
Grief (see Bereavement, Shock).
Grievance, unable to voice it
Grim, determined to survive.
Grudges held.

Guilt, so great it obstructs life..
***
H.
***
Half dead, apathetic.
Hallucinations (see a doctor).
Harmony craved.
Harsh,
Hate, simmering.
Hates other humans.
Head feels huge.
Hesitancy, uncertainty.
Highly strung.
Home, must go home.
Homesickness.
Hopelessness.
Hormone related hysteria.
Hostility, smoulders.
Humility and empathy absent.
Humiliation.
Hurry.
Hyperactive.
Hypersensitivity.
Hypochondria.
Hysteria.
Hurry.
Hysterical excitement.
***
I.
***
Identity lacking.

Idiocy.
Idiocy and moral depravity.
Ill-treatment from others leads to grief.
Imagination, stagnant..
Imposing love and rules on other people.
Impossible to please.
Impulses, violent, stammering.
Impulsive, aggressive, shuns people, checks things.
Incoherent.
Inconsolable.
Indecision.
Indecisive when alone.
Indifference to everything.
Indifference to loved ones.
Indignation.
Indolent.
Inert from exhaustion.
Inertia.
Influenced, too easily.
Initiative too low, sits and worries.
Injustice.
Insanity, brutal, kleptomania, avoids people, violent convulsions.
Insanity, fear that it is happening, in someone's head.
Insanity looming large.
Instability, extremes of emotion.
Insults, dwells on ancient ones.
Intellect overrules emotion and being human.
Interest in learning new things gone.
Interpersonal power craved.
Intimidated.

Irrational.
Irresolute.
Irritability if things seem slow.
Irritability with nausea, bearing down pains inside body.
Injures own skin.
Injustice, incensed with.
Insecure, emotionally.
Intolerant and critical of how other people do things.
***
J.
***
Jabbers mindlessly.
Jealousy.
Jubilant, too much, overdone.
Jumpy.
***
L.
***
Laughter, maniacal.
Laughter uncontrollable, followed by rage.
Laziness.
Learning from mistakes, impossible.
Let down.
Lethargy.
Liar.
Lies for attention.
Limbs, feels he has too many.
Limbs feel severed and scattered about.
Loathes self.
Longing, nostalgia.
Loquacity, too much.

Losses suffered.
Love, unable to give, blockage.
Lunatic behaviour in bursts, dangerous, mad.
***
M.
***
Malcontent.
Malicious.
Mania (insanity, nervous breakdown).
Manipulative, sly.
Martyr.
Matter-of-fact people.
Melancholia (see Depression, Winning, for information on the destructive wrath of melancholia).
Melancholic.
Memories, too sad.
Memory (fling and storing information).
Mental arguments.
Mental confusion (see Nervous breakdown).
Mental control, losing it.
Mental conversations, sometimes re-play continually.
Mental fatigue.
Mental troubles following sickness or injury.
Mind power gone.
Mind vacant.
Misfortunes of others affect her too much.
Mistakes, will not learn from.
Mixed up emotions.
Mixed feelings.
Monsters in the mind, patient bites and hits at them.
Mood swings.

Mood switches, restlessness.
Moon problems (full moon problems are common but rarely spoken about).
Mother hen consistently worrying about others.
Muddle-headed.
Murderous desires.
***
N.
***
Nags.
Names, calls things by wrong names.
Negatives, sees only.
Nervousness.
Nervous breakdown (see Discouragement, Apathy).
Nightmares.
Noise (hypersensitive to).
Noise, unable to tolerate.
Nosey.
***
O.
***
Obligations to loved-ones dropped.
Obstinate, heedless of others.
O.C.D. (Obsessive compulsive disorder).
Offended, takes offence too easily.
Omens.
Omnipotent, feels.
Opinions not allowed to be expressed.
Opportunity missed.
Order and efficiency.
Outbursts of rage.

Outraged.
Over-burdened.
Over-compliant.
Over-identification with the sufferings of others.
Over-stressed, keyed-up.
Over-sympathetic and over-critical.
Overwhelmed by life.
Overwrought, desperate to comply with requirements.
Own problems discussed in great depth.
***

P.
***

Pain, fear of.
Panic.
Paranoia.
Paranoid fears.
Past, lives in the past.
Past, unable to break from.
Peevish.
Peevish with homesickness and sleeplessness.
Perfection, demands it of himself and everyone else.
Perfection, standards too high.
Persecuted.
Perseverance not there.
Pessimistic.
Petulant.
Phobias (enduring fears, debilitating).
Plaintive speech.
Pleasure gone.
Plods on regardless.
Poise, lack of.

Pouting.
Preaches at others.
Precise, dominating.
Pre-occupied.
Pride (cannot endure failure, critical of others).
Procrastinates.
Public appearance, fear of.
Quietness, longs for.
***
R.
***
Rage.
Rage, apoplectic, sudden, with pulsating blood flow.
Rage, paroxysms.
Rage, uncontrolled.
Reclusive.
Red-faced rages.
Regression, into the past.
Regrets.
Relapses into old habits.
Release, longs for.
Religion, obsessive.
Remorse, filled with.
Repressed spirit.
Resentment.
Resentment, chronic, growing.
Resentful about petty politics.
Reserved.
Resigned, gives up.
Respect, deserves more.
Responsibility makes him flustered.

Restlessness, agitation, jumpiness, unbalanced.
Revenge.
Romantic, overdoes it.
Routine bound.
Routine, cannot stand it.
Rushes all the time.
Rut, in one.
Ruthlessness.
***
S.
***
Sadistic.
Sadism with cruelty, callousness, mistrust.
Sadness.
Sanctimonious.
Sanity, doubts own.
Satisfied, never.
Scathing comments.
Sceptical, of everything.
Schizophrenia, (see Nervous breakdown).
School phobia.
Scorned, feels scorned and mortified.
Screaming in fear.
Scruffy.
Secretive.
Security in relationships craved.
Self-confidence lacking.
Self-esteem undermined.
Self-image awful.
Self-opinionated.
Self-pity.

Self-reproach.
Self-reproach with persecution.
Self-righteous.
Self-sacrificial.
Self-trust, gone.
Senses depressed.
Sensitive, too quick to react, angry, impatient.
Sequence and order obsession.
Seriously, takes life too seriously.
Servile.
Setback, caused by something specific
Severe, inhuman.
Shame, deep.
Shiftless, lazy.
Shock and trauma (see Bereavement, Grief).
Shows off, noisily.
Shy.
Sleep disorders (see Insomnia).
Sleep disorders, intermittent, from internal conflicts.
Slow, feels slow and too big.
Slow thinking.
Sluggish and fat.
Smoking, after-effects.
Snobbish.
Solitude (craves for).
Someone behind.
Spaced out.
Speaking trouble, no idea what to say.
Spinning room, hammering in head.
Spiteful.
Spiteful but hard-working.

Squeamish.
Stagnated.
Stamina, emotional (none).
Stifled enjoyment.
Stifled people becoming introverted.
Strangers, afraid of.
Storms, fear of.
Struggle, unending.
Stubborn.
Stubborn and angry.
Stupidity, intolerant of.
Stupified.
Stupor.
Subservient.
Suffocating from people or talking.
Suicidal anguish.
Suicidal, to escape everything.
Suicidal.
Sulking.
Superstition, evil, ghosts.
Suppression of anger and annoyance.
Suppression of powerful, vital impulses.
Suspicious (of everyone, everything).
Suspicious of everything and everyone.
Switches of emotion.
Sympathy, craves.
***

T.
***

Tactless.
Tantrums in children and adults (see Temper).

Task too huge, dreams recede.
Tearful, crying.
Tearful, sentimental.
Tears, suddenly, unexpected.
Tedium, too much.
Temper, sudden and hot.
Tentative.
Terrors (night) (see Panic, Fear).
Theatrical.
Thick-skinned.
Thinking unclear, ineffective.
Thinking very difficult, apathetic, lazy.
Thoughts, of past.
Thunder (terror) (see Storms)..
Thwarted, constantly.
Tics.
Ties, old ties too strong.
Tight clothing, aversion to, talks non-stop.
Time, no conception.
Timid and slow, superstitious.
Tired, with life.
Tolerance, none.
Touchy, ugly, dissatisfied.
Touch, aversion to.
Touch, fear of.
Tongue-tied.
Trapped, stagnated, unable to get going.
Trembles with fear, needs to urinate.
Trivialities assume huge proportions.
Trivialities obsess the mind.
Trust absent.

Turbulence of the mind.
Turmoil of emotions.
Two selves, near death.
***
U.
***
Ugly behaviour, dread.
Ugly, thinks one is.
Unappreciated, not valued.
Understanding of events poor.
Uneasy, all the time.
Unfettered by conventions.
Unhappiness, no reason, just a cloud descending.
Unreasonable.
Unreliable, lacks courage, not a stable person.
Unresponsive.
Unsuccessful after long efforts.
Unsettled, cannot settle down to tasks of life.
***
V.
***
Vacant.
Vacilatory.
Vengeful.
Vertigo.
Vexed, ugly behaviour.
Victimised, feels.
Victimised, resentful.
Vulnerable, threatened.
***
W.

***

Walks great distances.
Weeps, for no reason.
Weepy, clingy, whiney people.
Welfare of others a constant worry.
Wild, irrational ideas and uncontrolled thoughts.
Will subjugated.
Winning.
Worry.
Wrong, everything.
***

Y.
***

Yielding.
***

Z.
***

Zombie.
***

5. Selection of material for this book.
***

The complete selection of material is based on many decades of observation and study. It reflects an interest in the human organism, as a microcosm, with all its intricacies and foibles. Fundamental to all this, is the realisation that the body, mind and spirit form a fully interactional and integral unit. It is not possible, except conceptionally and erroneously, to isolate any disorder or facet of its being, and to imagine that it exists alone.

The most important consideration is the emotional component, without which very little is possible. Next comes the mental component, followed by the physical, which includes diseases and injuries.

This book is about the emotional and mental aspects of treatment and health.
***

6. Introduction (remedy dosage and selection).
***

Homeopathy has helped millions and millions of people, animals, and birds around the world for hundreds of years. It is a wonderful form of healing, with no side-effects or dangers involved.

Dosage is effected by popping the pillule/powder/liquid into the mouth of the patient, preferably under the tongue, where it is quickly absorbed. The remedy may be dissolved in drinking water and shaken violently for a minute, or in extreme cases mixed with food.

Selection of a remedy for chronic (long-term) disorders, ideally involves an analysis of the patient's emotions, mental processes, modalities (what makes it better or worse), cravings and aversions, sidedness of the symptoms, family and personal history, medical history, physical problems, other factors and the presenting (complained about) symptoms. We are not always able to establish this with all people, because of time restraints, incomplete remedy information, or interpersonal factors, so frequently use only the presenting symptom, which is sometimes but not always insufficient. However, if a presenting symptom is acute (of sudden appearance), then it is often sufficient, especially in the case of emotion-related disorders such as loss of confidence, loss of motivation, depression, anticipation anxiety, exam fears, jealousy, obsessions, mania, bipolar problems, trauma, or other mental or emotional disorders.

This book is a very brief guide to rapid or emergency prescribing, mostly inadequate for complete professional prescribing, although of great use in emergencies or at home. It should be supplemented, where possible, with consultation of a good Materia Medica such as Boericke, where more information for each remedy can be found, and a better choice made. The more points in the remedy that match the patient's symptoms, the better the chances of cure are.

An understanding of dosage is important. Stop the dosage the moment there is any improvement, and re-dose if improvement stops. In a crisis you may need to administer six doses in a day (but then stop or change remedies), but normally one remedy may do the trick, or one dose per day for a few days. You need to observe the effects and make your own judgement. If improvement occurs and you continue the dose, the effect may cease permanently. Some remedies may act days later. Big or small patients need the same dose. Use your savvy.

Strength of dose? I suggest 30C or higher (possibly 200C) for emotional and mental problems, but others may also work. Try the suggested remedies one at a time until one works. Some organisms do not respond to any medications, but most of them do. Low-strength remedies like D6, or anything lower than 30C, are likely to act more quickly, but mostly only on physical symptoms, leaving mental-emotional problems untouched. They also leave the system more rapidly.

Common maladies are listed in alphabetical order below. It is a good idea to have a separate note book to record all treatments and results. Fairly common remedies are suggested with as much overlap as possible so you do not need to buy too many to keep in stock. There are thousands more than are mentioned here. Run your eye down the bold listings, to rapidly locate the ailment, followed by possible suitable remedies. Later a proper repertorisation of each remedy should be carried out, if possible, for better results

It is strongly recommended that you carefully read through all the notes here, and familiarize yourself with the layout, as in an emergency people fail to think clearly and may not be able to locate the most appropriate remedy. Browse the book regularly and become familiar with everything in it.

Bach's Flower Remedies can be most effective, and are in themselves complex and complete. They work on the body via the emotional system, and are covered in this book.

Names of remedies are the same the world over, in Latin, which is very useful. Shortened forms may differ e.g. Bryonia may be Br, Bry, Bryon.

***

7. Vis Medicatrix Naturae.
***

This refers to the natural healing power within any body. It is the ability to recognise and repel invaders and repair damage caused by any source. Sometimes this ability can be impaired to various degrees. It is difficult to fully define where disease begins and ends, but when the natural healing powers are not properly functional, then a state of disease is presumed to exist.

There are two major forms of medicine available to assist the body in regaining its natural powers. The one is the medicine of contraries, e.g. where to medicate for pain, a pain-killer is administered. The other is the medicine of Similars, where a substance which causes the same symptoms in a healthy patient, as the patient to be treated exhibits, is administered in miniscule form, and it jogs the body into repelling the problem. The dose is so infinitesimal that not even one single atom is administered, only the nuclear imprint of it, with the substance diluted millions of times. A complete atom might kill the patient at times, since the substances used are sometimes deadly poisonous in undiluted form. However, in diluted form they are completely harmless, and have no effect whatsoever on a healthy body.

Homeopathy is based on the administration of the Simillimum, or the Similar, and is totally safe with no side-effects. Once the Vis Medicatrix Naturae has been activated, the body often heals all its own problems without further assistance. Naturally this makes very little money for the remedy manufacturers, and would put many orthodox medicine manufacturers out of business, so consequently the orthodox establishment sometimes goes to extreme lengths to try to discredit homeopathy. Imagine a manufacturer of childrens' medicines (among others in a huge range of products), which sells millions of doses per day, making an average of one dollar per dose, per day for many years, per child. Considering a homeopathic dose might cure the problem, you can imagine what gigantic stakes are really at play here. Of course this is not the case with all manufacturers nor all orthodox medicines, but I am sure you can see the principle. Homeopathy can not cause depressions, suicidal tendencies and other side-effects. It also cannot cure many potentially fatal diseases that orthodox medicine can treat with various invasive techniques and emergency procedures, blood transfusions, x-rays and similar. Assess the strength of your patient's Vis Medicatrix Naturae (people can be very good at assessing their patient's Vital Force), and decide which path to follow. Hopefully this book will provide you with some assistance in the choice of treatment for emotional and mental requirements in humans, and possibly also the treatment of animals and birds.

Hippocrates, the famous Greek physician, taught that medicines merely created the correct conditions for the individual's natural healing power, the Vis Medicatrix Naturae, to restore the balance of the system, and enable it to remove the symptoms of illness.

The Vis Medicatrix Naturae is inextricably interwoven with the concept of the Vital Force, the activation of which, by the administration of homeopathic remedies, leads to recovery from various ills and injuries. The natural healing power within the person, is powered by the

Vital Force, or "chi" or "prana", which is an urgent, driven, powerful energy, sometimes dormant and sometimes active. Specially trained people can summon or activate this force at will. The natural healing power is also evidenced in ways which show its presence, other than in healing. For instance a small woman is suddenly able to carry a heavy child at a run for a long distance to escape danger. Sometimes this natural healing power is activated by external forces, and other times by the system itself, but when it is not in action as it should be, it can be stimulated into action by homeopathic remedies. Also by focus and concentration, self-hypnosis, hypnosis, meditation, acupuncture and yoga, and other complementary systems, the Vital force or natural healing powers can be jolted into curing illnesses and other problems. It is something akin to a supercharger of bodily abilities and mental fortitude.

The Vis Medicatrix Naturae is not visible to the eye, except in its manifestations of energy and healing in a person, and is in itself a major energy field. It is also present in animals, birds, fish, plants, trees and living entities.

Some current speculation regards the natural healing power as a possible bioplasm of ionised particles, held in proximity to each other by energy. It is thought to affect growth and development as it effects repairs on the system. It may be an energy double of the physical body, tightly connected, and interlaced with all its aspects. Its stimulation leads to recovery from illness and injury. The healing force effects changes in mind, body and emotions.

The healing power of the body, is an inherent ability to establish, maintain and restore good health. Nature heals through the response of the Vis Medicatrix Naturae, which is an ordered and intelligent process. The homeopath's remedy facilitates and augments this process, to act and identify and remove obstacles to health and recovery, and to support the creation of a healthy internal and external environment.

First described in Western medicine by Hippocrates, the Vis Medicatrix Naturae, is also referred to as "chi" in Chinese Medicine, "prana" in Ayurveda, and "Vital Force" in homeopathy. When alive, the Vis Medicatrix Naturae enables humans and other living beings to resist entropy and decay, unlike inanimate objects that are not subject to these effects at the same rapid rate that living beings are. Creating treatment plans that harness the healing power of nature, that incorporate dietary and lifestyle improvements, that employ the least invasive, least harmful and most effective therapies, is the art, the heart and the essence of homeopathic medicine.

***

What is Homeopathy?

***

8. Definition of Homeopathy.

***

Homeopathy is a system of medicine based on the principle of treating like with like. Its name derives from the Greek words "homoios" (like) and "pathos" (suffering). It is designed to restore the human being to a state of equilibrium, and therefore health, by treating the causes of illness, acute and chronic disease, accidents, befallments and acute mistunements, traumas, emotional and mental disturbances, rather than symptoms. By the administration of a pathogenic substance, which in itself produces the same symptoms in a healthy person, as the patient has, the organism (human being usually) is "kick-started" into curing itself. Homeopathy is characterised by this principle, which is termed the "similia law" or "law of similars".

Homeopathy is holistic in nature, treating the constitution, or whole person, rather than symptoms in isolation. Remedies used are the tiniest possible doses of natural substances, like plants, animals, insects and minerals. Homeopathy frees patients from disease symptoms, and restores inner harmony, improving energy, work, relationships and life. Homeopathy stimulates the Vital Force within the patient, which regulates and repairs and heals the system.

***

9. The two main principles of homeopathy.
***

a) The first principle (Law of Similars) initially states that every active substance that acts on the functions of the body provokes a set of symptoms characteristic to that substance in a healthy, sensitive body. An example of this is coffee, which causes an acceleration of the heart rate, increased urine output, nervous excitation, insomnia and a heightening of the senses. Now the principle states that any substance which can make you ill can also cure you. If it can produce the symptoms of the disease in a healthy body, then it can also cure those symptoms in a sick body.

Every diseased body exhibits a range of symptoms characteristic to that illness. An example of this is mental overexertion, which produces a heightened heart rate, insomnia, excitability, a racing mind, increased sensitivity to noise or light and touch.

These two phenomena are the basics used to identify a cure, which will be demonstrated by the disappearance of the symptoms, brought about by the prescription of a low or infinitesimal dose of a substance that would produce similar symptoms in a healthy person. Therefore "Coffea" in homeopathic dose, would cure the above patient. This is a demonstration of the Law of Similars, being the principle of "let like be treated by like", or similia similibus curentur. The symptom profile must always be matched with the remedy profile, as one is treating the patient, not the disease. Each patient will probably demonstrate some different symptom profiles for the same disease, and so will not necessarily be treated with the same remedy as everyone else, and each patient should be treated as an individual, needing individualised treatment, rather than being grouped by disease for a remedy e.g. giving everyone with a sore throat the same remedy (which would be homeopathically wrong but perhaps correct for orthodox medicine). Unless the Law of Similars is correctly applied, the treatment will be worthless.

b)   The second principle is the Law of Potentised Remedies. Extreme dilution enhances the curative properties of a substance, while eliminating side-effects. Furthermore, in conventional medicine, as the concentration is decreased, so the medicine becomes less effective (potent), until a point is reached where it stops working, whereas in homeopathic medicine with each dilution (and succussion, or violent shake) it gains in potency, and this is the basis of homeopathic Potentised Remedies. This is what separates homeopathy from orthodox medicine, and upsets those rigid minds of critics who cannot conceive of something beyond their preconceptions. In homeopathy the energy levels present in the remedies are what promote the cure, and not the actual amount of the substance. As all remedies have many facets, and can produce various symptoms in healthy people, it is possible and preferable to prescribe only a single correct remedy at a time. By doing this its precise effect can be observed, and the homeopath can proceed further with other remedies for stubborn or newly-emerging other symptoms. Furthermore, it is commonly felt that the smallest possible dose required to nudge the healing process into action, is the best. This is in keeping with the highly diluted and therefore highly potentised homeopathic remedy that homeopaths use.

***
10. The term, "the similar".
***

The "similar" refers to the homeopathic remedy, which when administered to a healthy body, will cause that body to exhibit the same symptoms as the patient is experiencing. The appropriate use of processed substances similar to the disease, can restore a sick body to a state of balance, and therefore health. Diseases are therefore shown to succumb to substances which cause a similar ailment, hence the word "similar" to describe each substance. Hahnemann suggested that this is because nature will not allow two similar diseases to exist in the body at the same time, so the newly introduced one will push the old one out. Each patient does not respond to a "similar" in the same way as every other patient, and because each patient exhibits a different response, an entire "symptom picture" of each patient needs to be found, so that the selected "similar" will match the patient's individual needs in as many ways as possible, and not simply become a general hit-or-miss remedy. A "similar" may be identified by careful use of a Materia Medica, once the patient's profile has been established. A good Materia Medica lists all symptoms a substance may cause in a healthy person, and therefore a study of substances to find one which most perfectly matches the patient's symptoms, will expose the closest "similar" for appropriate administration.

A "similar" should be selected on the basis of causing similar symptoms (in a healthy body), to the patient's symptoms, in as many fields as possible. These include characteristics (e.g. fidgets), general symptoms (such as attitude, outlook, reactions to the disease and other matters of life), mentals (emotional makeup, fears, phobias, drives, introversions etc), modalities (all matters which aggravate or ameliorate the situation, like weather, season, body position, time of day, eating, water, keeping still, and numerous others), likes and dislikes (cravings and aversions), physical characteristics (expression, walk, posture, appearance, skin, hair etc), disease tendencies of the past and present, family history (reason for, and time of deaths), patient's history (trauma etc), emotional tendencies such as doubt, agoraphobia etc.). The better the remedy matches the patient profile the more effectively it will cure the patient. A homeopath should always seek the most perfect, or closest "similar", starting with the mentals, then going on to the reactions to the world, then cravings and aversions and then the particulars to that patient's body, broadly speaking (Kent).

The above information is sometimes termed differently, and Hahnemann, the great German physician, termed all the patient information the "symptom picture". The symptoms induced in healthy people by substances (drugs), he called the "drug picture". The more similar the "symptom picture" and the "drug picture" are, the more likely the treatment is to be successful, and the stronger the likelihood that the remedy and the disease will cancel each other out. It is always necessary to find the patient's symptoms first, before matching them to different remedies so as to find the most appropriate one.

***

11. Acute and Chronic conditions.
***

An acute condition comes on quickly and often departs quickly. It can be caused by infection or temporary imbalance of the system, or stress, injury, overexertion, trauma, an accident, a death, etc. Infections causing acute conditions can be colds, coughs or bacterial or viral infections. Acute also refers to bruising, bleeding, convulsions or loss of consciousness. In acute conditions that the homeopath cannot cope with, a doctor should be called. Orthodox medicine has symptom drugs for acute conditions, such as anti-spasm, anti-coagulant, stings, and so on. Acute conditions are new and recent, not deep-seated, and sometimes clear on their own. Some can be fatal, such as meningitis, nephritis or pneumonia. Acute diseases have the distinct phases of incubation (no symptoms), acute phase (the symptoms surface), and the convalescent phase showing strong improvement. Home remedies ease the pain and speed up recovery in many acute illnesses such as food poisoning, 'flu and childrens' illnesses, ensuring there are no complications.

Acute states are departures from the usual state and can be physical or mental/emotional.

A chronic condition is quite different, showing a history of various complaints, with deep underlying causes, recurrences, lowered vitality and steadily declining general health. People feel unwell yet medical tests reveal nothing. The origins may be chronic diseases. Chronic diseases mistune the living organism with small unnoticed beginnings, and the state of health declines, steadily until death. The Vital Force is unable to stop this as it increases, leading to final destruction of the organism.

There is an idea, incorrect, among certain people, that the word "acute" refers to the sharpness or degree of severity of a complaint. This is not accurate, as a chronic complaint may be much more painful or severe than an acute one, in some instances.

Unlike acute diseases, a chronic disease does not take a predictable course, and one cannot say how long it will last. It can even stem from the complications following an acute disease. Examples of chronic disease are heart problems, cancer and mental illness. Some may be caused by chemicals in food and in the air, overuse of orthodox medicines (e.g. painkillers) and general environmental pollution, either chemical, noise, too many people, or other.

An acute illness may be infectious so the patient may need to keep away from other people. In some cases only rest may be needed for people to recover, or perhaps, relaxation, fresh air, good food and some pampering. A chronic state is probably not infectious and will probably become worse irrespective of rest or diet and pampering. Acute cases can be caused by simple exhaustion and being run down, but chronic ones are deep-seated, arising from infection or miasms passed down from previous generations.

People suffering from acute conditions can usually pinpoint the problem e.g. a very sore joint, or a sore throat, while in chronic cases the patient probably suffers from a host of different symptoms (seemingly unrelated as far as the patient is concerned). Treatment for acute symptoms is usually specific and may be aimed at soft tissue, with short-lasting low potency remedies. Chronic conditions may need years of treatment or a long time to recover, with the use of high potency remedies, or constitutional remedies.

Acute conditions may require frequent taking of remedies even down to every fifteen minutes or so in extremis (e.g. head injury) while chronic treatments may require a single remedy taken once, which acts for months or years. Acute conditions may clear very rapidly, perhaps even within the hour, while chronic ones may take years.

It is very simple to repertorise for an acute condition as it often is a case of single symptom repertorising, but chronic conditions may require many hours of sleuthing and hard work to identify symptoms, construct a good symptom picture, and then match it to remedies to try to find the most complete match.

Trauma rooms and outpatient's departments in hospitals, usually deal with acute situations, like falls down steps. Chronic ones have gone on for a long time and do not call for sudden intervention, like oxygen, operations, pain killers, sedatives etc, except at the end.

There are certain acute conditions which require urgent medical attention and where a doctor should be consulted. Homeopaths can make these situations more comfortable, but should not attempt to deal with them. They are neck and back injuries, chest and abdominal wounds, protruding or broken bones, burns that are not small, cyanosis (turning blue), chest pains, unconsciousness, severe head injury, seizures, difficulty in breathing, shock for more than an hour, bleeding more than just a little bit. In chronic conditions there is not this sudden trauma, but a slow insidious ingress of problems over a long period, perhaps decades.

Some common acute situations are injuries, food poisoning, insect or snake or dog bites, burns or scalds, gastro-intestinal problems, cuts and abrasions, fright. These are quite different to chronic situations like cancers, rheumatism, arthritis etc.

One source says a rule of thumb for determining whether a condition is acute or chronic, is whether it arrives and clears within six months or not.   Perhaps this is too simplistic a model.

Mental and emotional disorders are frequently tied up with other disorders, possibly causing them or being caused by them. Some disorders of the mind are acute and some are chronic, and some can be both, as in anger from childhood and anger with the boss.

***

12. Fundamental Disease.
***

This concept originates with the possibility that all manifestations of illness (symptoms) are merely indicators of a fundamental disease within the system. This disease affects, from within, the body and mind of the sufferer. The subtle body is affected and unable to tune all the aspects of the Vital Force adequately, so as to ensure vibrant good health. Because of this mistunement, different problems and symptoms appear at different times. The symptoms are an indicator of the fundamental disease. Symptoms are not seen in isolation, as with orthodox medicine, but can be collected and listed, and will point to the fundamental cause of them all. Fundamental diseases collect in the body sometimes, like walled off capsules, emerging from time to time when the Vital Force, weakened by the fundamental disease, is not able to maintain the walls adequately. Sometimes these manifestations are described as rings (like in an onion), with each ring being a burned out or suppressed disease, waiting to show a symptom, when the fundamental disease weakens the Vital Force sufficiently. They can be caused by, or brought into existence by various things such as drugs or antibiotics (suppression) or by trauma, mental or emotional (death, stress) or physical causes (motor accident). Each one leaves a residue or imprint. In a healthy body they may never emerge again, but in a weakened one they may emerge in different forms from time to time. A wart, for instance, when cut off, may cause other symptoms to emerge, such as asthma, as they could all be caused by the same fundamental disease.

Suppression or removing of a symptom (which the system is using as a valve to cope with the disease) may increase the internal pressure, resulting in the emergence of other symptoms.   It may be better to treat the fundamental disease with constitutional remedies, than to treat local symptoms and leave the fundamental disease untouched and active. Activity on individual symptoms, may activate or stimulate the fundamental disease.

Ultimately, a very complicated interaction among the layers of disease, may arise from interference with individual symptoms, resulting in multi-system chronic disease.   A whole range of symptoms may then simultaneously arise, and defy all efforts to deal with them. An example might be the arthritis, skin problems and emotional changes of rheumatoid arthritis, or otherwise catarrh, migraine and colitis.

Hahnemann found that the disposition of a patient was a decidedly characteristic symptom which should chiefly determine the selection of a homeopathic remedy. He also noted that a complete picture of an individual required an understanding of the primary, latent and secondary states of fundamental miasms. In his early days he noted that some patients responded not at all, or less and less, to remedies, indicating that a fundamental disease was operating and perhaps causing all the chronic symptoms. For twelve years he sought the fundamental cause of the symptoms which plagued some patients, and in various great works he concluded that chronic miasms could be responsible.   One can have a number of miasms all contributing to disease and various symptoms, and they can be a fundamental cause, and also an obstruction to remedies. In short, they form a sort of fundamental disease, or set of diseases, within patients suffering from chronic diseases.

In order to discover a fundamental cause, whether it be a miasm or not, the investigation should include all ascertainable information about the physical state of the patient, his moral and intellectual character, occupation, mode of living and habits, social and domestic relations, age, sexual function and everything else. Since a fundamental disease will affect all of this, it can also cause various symptoms.

Fundamental diseases can be slow, insidious, with a gradual onset and slow progression. Complex pathologies result, and premature old age and death follow. They damage the Vital Force, the immune system, and the constitution.

So while it may not be completely possible to describe what a fundamental disease really is, the totality of symptoms can make us aware of its existence, and point to appropriate remedies. This has been a very brief description of the fundamental disease and fundamental cause. It is intended to demonstrate that not all disorders can be treated quickly and simply. A qualified and experienced homeopath may need to be consulted.

***

13. Duration of remedy action and repeat dosage.
***

In homeopathy, there is a school of thought which suggests the homeopath take some time and effort, in order to select the correct simillimum.   After the simillimum is administered, everyone should wait patiently (the patient should have been appraised of the mode of operation of a homeopathic remedy), and in due course the Vital Force should respond appropriately and the symptoms, after a possible aggravation, should diminish or disappear. Although there are different durations of expected action, each case is individual, and a close watch should be kept to see if and when the action begins, and how long it endures for.   Once a remedy has had its effect, even if it is still within the expected duration of time, and the effect has worn off or run its course and is no more, then the remedy can be repeated if the symptoms remain the same. If they have changed (symptoms from the outer ring of the onion model have been removed and new ones exposed underneath), then another remedy, or a different potency might be indicated.

In the case of no action from the remedy, one might consider that an inappropriate remedy has been prescribed, or a wrong potency, or perhaps a miasm is stopping any action.   However, if you take Arsenicum album as an example, there is an expected action of between sixty and ninety days, leaving a full thirty days of uncertainty and a margin on either side for individual differences, stronger Vital Force etc. If a remedy has had its effect and this has not been recorded or observed, then the patient might wait for ninety days or more wondering if the remedy is going to cure him, when in fact a repeat dose may have been called for.

If a remedy is working, a repeat dose may stop the action, or slow it.   If the remedy does not work within the expected time, it could be the wrong potency or the wrong remedy.   A new remedy, or a different potency might be required, or increased frequency of doses.   Alternatively, the patient's constitution may be different to usual patients and this may change the time spans of the remedies.

So it seems that although a remedy's expected action of duration should be understood and borne in mind, by both the patient and the homeopath, it should not be strictly adhered to, but rather the action of the first dose should be monitored and used as the guide for whether a repeat dose is necessary, within the expected duration time of that remedy.

Fundamentally, after a homeopathic dose, no new one should be administered until the effect of the first one has ceased.   Patients may improve after the first dose, and need doses less and less frequently.   Alternatively there may be improvement after each dose, and doses may need to be brought closer to each other until cure is effected.   A greater potency may be the answer in that case.   One can "plus" (dissolve tablets in water, shake vigorously, and have spoonfuls at perhaps hourly intervals if the response is good but short-lived).   One can agitate the water to possibly increase or maintain effectiveness.   If the remedy stops working the remedy should be reviewed and perhaps a new one tried.   On rare occasions the remedy could have died in the container and the patient and homeopath could wait forever.

Vigorous illness responds to remedies vigorously. Slow or sluggish illnesses take longer to respond. Fast ones may need treatment several times an hour while they are acute, and symptoms may also change. Usually the more severe the illness, the simpler the diagnosis is. Incorrect remedies will not harm people. Slow illnesses may be treated once every day. "Average" illnesses may need treatment three to eight times a day, diminishing in number. Colds etc can be treated three times a day. When one is unsure and cannot find a guideline, it might be worth simply guessing, so as to get the treatment into action. It is better to try something, as it cannot harm the patient, than to do nothing because of being unsure. The remedy must be stopped when the patient is cured.

As can be seen above, the expected duration of the effect of the remedy may not always be taken into account, especially in acute cases, and dosage may be dependent upon the individual's actual reaction to the remedy.

***

14. Constitutional types and remedies.
***

Why have healers been keen on working out constitutional types?
***

Healers have tried to categorise patients. By taking into account physical characteristics, emotional and mental tendencies, strengths and weaknesses, and their modalities, they have tools for working out the state of balance or imbalance within the individual. This way the healer can determine appropriate healing remedies. By analysing the patient the healer can construct a picture of the patient, which in homeopathic terms is called the "constitutional picture", and which reveals the "constitutional type" of the patient. The selected remedy is chosen because it matches the temperament, character, outlook and features, historical tendencies and symptom patterns of the patient and is said to be the "constitutional remedy" for that patient.

Constitutional prescribing seeks a simplified, boxed and complete method of determining the most appropriate remedy, by trying to analyse and identify the type, then matching it to the symptoms of various remedies until, if possible, the exact match is found. This match will be the correct constitutional remedy and should cure all mistunements within the system, provided the match is comprehensive enough. It is far more comprehensive (in homeopathy) than the simple allopathic or psychological, broad spectrum type of labelling we find, such as "infection of the stomach" or "schizophrenia", which indicate a possible remedy for many different states of the same disease. Rather, numerous symptoms are exposed, and used to identify the constitutional type. Constitutional remedies are also used for maintenance of equilibrium and health, and keeping the entire system in tune. Constitutional remedies are completely personal to the patient and not generalized, in homeopathy.

It is very convenient for any healer to identify a constitutional type, so that all his further healing can be based on that model, although it may not be accurate. I have been reading about one healer who identifies all his human constitutional types by a rapid glance at their finger nails, and prescribes without delay on this basis, which to my way of thinking is over-simplified.

Numerous books have been written to assist in the discovery of constitutional types, or "bodymind homeopathic personalities". Some of the authors are P. Bailley, E.C. Whitmont, R. Sankaran, P. Chappell and many more. Some combine psychology with homeopathy, others combine paediatrics, others allopathy, and some look at up to three hundred remedies in depth.

There are literally constellations of various types of constitutional "typing" going back into history, based on various aspects of humans, such as morphology, physiology and psychology. Galen proposed his famous sanguine, melancholic, choleric and phlegmatic types. Kretshmer identified pyknics, asthenics, dysplastics, ectomorphic and endomorphic types, which have been taught at universities for decades. To me they all seem over-simplified, as humans have combinations of many things within them and all prescribing needs to be specific to each person. So far, I have not found any similar, and convincing, systems within the non-human kingdoms, although one cannot discount the possibility that in the future some usable "typing" may be developed by those healing birds, animals, fish and reptiles.

In homeopathy, a time came when Hahnemann found that using symptoms alone was not always sufficient to prescribe an effective remedy. He realized that the transitory symptom picture was only a part of what was required by the homeopath. This led to an evaluation of the character, the life situation, the living habits, the likes and dislikes, social and domestic relations, sex and sexual tendencies and everything else, all of which can be used to determine the constitution of the patient, which assists in the selection of the most useful remedy.

Some homeopaths say, look at the appearance of the patient first, then the mental and emotional aspects, followed by the physical weaknesses, then try to find the closest constitutional type. Then look at what they came about, perhaps stomach aches, and repertorise stomach ache remedies, to find several, of which one should be the constitutional remedy, which is what to prescribe.

Korean medicine traditionally identifies four basic constitutional types, Ayurvedic (simplified) three types, and other systems sometimes have more, but homeopathy has hundreds of constitutional types, being very thorough and personalised.

Once a homeopath has an overview of the patient's constitutional type, he is in a position to try to match it to the remedy which has the same profile in as many symptoms as possible. This means looking at everything about the patient, and finding, the remedy which will act upon the very core of the patient. This should activate the

Vital Force in such a way that the entire system is brought back into balance and harmonised, in a manner which radiates outwards from the core, affecting first the outer ring of symptoms, and then moving inwards, casing brief flare-up and then cure of each symptom. The most recent symptom would react first, followed by the next most recent, and so on, until, all would be gone. One can compare the rings with layers like an onion has, and The Law of Cure states that the newest ones (outer) are disposed of first, followed by the others.

Of course, a deep-acting constitutional remedy, should ideally be administered in a high potency, but locally-focussed remedies (for tissue damage, breaks etc), should be in low potencies.

In constitutional prescribing, we are using the deep acting high potency remedies to act directly upon the subtle or ethereal body to restore harmony. Because the "rings" of symptoms may stretch back from many years, or decades, this could take a long time, perhaps years. There could be brief recurrences of old illnesses, aggravations of current acute illnesses, and in certain cases more than one constitutional remedy might be indicated. Indian and Greek schools tend to favour more than one such remedy. Classical constitutional or Kentian prescribers (called Unicists in Europe), like to prescribe only one remedy at a time, so they can see which one is affecting what. They believe that ideally one remedy should encapsulate the entire patient. The Pluralists may prescribe several at a time and are sometimes termed complex prescribers, and they mix remedies. I believe this approach should be made with great care as the effects may be unpredictable or unwanted. Complex remedies, such as calcarea carbonica, already consist of thousands of chemicals.

Various medicine systems identify "types" and try to link up physical characteristics, and emotional profiles, strengths and weaknesses etc to see where the internal balance is impaired. In Ayurvedic the three humours join at birth to produce seven constitutional types. In Islamic medicine, four humours combine to produce eleven constitutional types. In homeopathy we analyse the interaction of physical and mental features to find the profile of the patient and thereby identify the correct remedy. Hence we arrive at the "Arsenic types" etc. There are numerous types and numerous remedies with no strict categorisation. We match the patient profile to the remedy profile to cure the patient.

A constitutional picture may reveal a homeopathic type. Symptoms and reactions present a recognisable pattern of general physical, particular and mental/emotional symptoms e.g. a calcarea carbonica type is likely to be overweight, fair-haired, fearful and lacking in confidence, perspire on the head when asleep and crave boiled eggs. The pattern correlates with the picture of the remedy and is verified by clinical experience. Identifying a type is useful in the objective understanding of a pattern, but because of individualisation the remedy selected may differ from that of the classical type. An acute symptom may hide the details of the type, or the constitutional picture. A good homeopath should take into account the patient's type, nature and symptoms. A constitutional remedy sometimes results in an aggravation (intensification) of some symptoms before the patient starts feeling better. Cure is not measured by symptom-relief alone, but by how you feel physically emotionally and mentally. Constitutional remedies may result in anything from a very slow to a very swift cure.

What we are trying to do in constitutional prescribing, can be well demonstrated by using a Lycopodium Type, in human beings, as an example. These constitutional types tend to be thin, spare, nervous and have pains on the right hand side, appearing self-confident, but having low self-confidence, and being flatulent and feeling full after small meals. The homeopath will study the patient to determine the constitutional type, and will not merely study the disease. Constitutional types have physical characteristics, emotional profiles, strengths and weaknesses, and the homeopath can spot the internal imbalances and treat them. A type is a combination of physical and psychological factors, and the way they interact together and with their environs. The homeopath seeks a matching remedy profile. He may spot an Arsenicum, Phosphorus or Sulphur type etc and treat the constitution accordingly. In Ayurvedic or in Islamic medicine there are fixed types, but in homeopathy we acknowledge numerous combinations and seek matching remedy profiles. Thus it can be quite a complicated undertaking to successfully locate a patient's constitutional type, and more especially so if the patient cannot speak.

Constitutional types are prone to certain corresponding diseases, and constitutional remedies may cure these diseases and stop their constant recurrence, while orthodox treatment simply walls off certain manifestations (symptoms) of the disease, which will then emerge as different things. Constitutional remedies are normally administered in 30C or higher potencies perhaps monthly, although on occasion they may be given in lower potencies daily.

When a system is at ease, or in balance, it is able to detect and overcome harmful influences. When it fails to do this, it finds itself no longer at ease, but in a state of dis-ease. This can become worse and embed itself for life, and even kill the host. It can be emotional and/or physical and root causes can be multiple e.g. a fall, emotional stress, a loss of protectors, an illness, or any of many others, which have resulted in the constitution no longer being able to heal itself. A constitutional remedy can restore the vigour of the Vital Force and stimulate it to cure the disease.

Homeopathic remedies have a wide range of action in certain disease states, and certain constitutions have a tendency towards certain illnesses. These do not include acute problems like accidents, psychological traumas etc. The physical symptoms of the disease can be modified by orthodox medicines to create the illusion of healing, although the chronic disease is really only being temporarily walled off and will re-emerge in different forms, only to be shot away by anti-biotics, to reappear elsewhere. The fundamental disease, mistunements or imbalances, stay in place.

By prescribing a constitutional remedy which matches the profile of the patient, one is prescribing a deep acting historical remedy which works on disease from long ago, right up the most recent, enabling the Vital Force to recognise and cure the problems.
***

15. Administering remedies, dose and potency.
***

The homeopathic remedy should only be taken until it starts working, and then stopped, or otherwise unexpected symptoms may appear, or the remedy may be reflected by the body and not work at all. In any event the absolute minimum dose should be taken for the minimum amount of time. Homeopathic remedies in shops have recommended dosages on the labels, and this is ridiculous, in view of what I have said above. The important factor is the frequency, and not the potency of the dosage, and doses must be stopped when improvement is seen.

For people who may be allergic to lactose pillules, it is advisable to select other forms of tablet or liquid form of the remedy. However, pills are probably preferable to powders, granules and liquids, easy to store and take without having to sterilize droppers.

Tablets should be handled as little as possible, and then flicked into the mouth under the tongue or into the cheek. Those which are dropped or roll away somewhere should not be put back into the bottle but should be thrown away, as they may be contaminated with undesirable substances, or may have had their medicine rubbed off their surface. A patient may touch his own tablets, although not recommended, but other patients should not touch anyone else's remedy. One's own bugs may be acceptable to one's own system but another patient's may not be.

Tablets should be dissolved under the tongue so they can be absorbed into the system without being mixed up with too much food, other toxic substances, or stomach acids, which might make them less effective. In the case of very hard tablets, it is acceptable to chew them a little first before dissolving them under the tongue.

One tablet or dose is sufficient and gives the same benefit as two or more, no matter how big the patient is. If you struggle to get the patient to take the dose, then dissolve it in the patient's water, or at worst crush a few and put them in a little food, but food may contaminate their efficacy. In a poultry shed when treating chickens, for instance, it is best to dissolve a few tablets in the water.

If a patient spits out the tablets, they can be dissolved in a little spring water, stirred vigorously, and given in sips from time to time, with vigorous stirring or shaking to re-potentise the remedy fully each time. An unconscious patient can have this rubbed onto the lips, for the remedy to work.

Storage of remedies must be in cool dark areas (e.g. a drawer or cupboard), free of any strong smells or volatile substances which might inactivate them. They must be distanced from mobile phones, radiation of any sort (microwaves), direct sunlight and moisture which could damage or inactivate their efficiency. Inimical (hostile) to homeopathic remedies, may be household cleaners, perfumed cosmetics and toiletries and mints. Certain aromatherapy oils such as peppermint, camphor, eucalyptus, rosemary, thyme and lavender, may antidote or neutralise the remedies.

If new symptoms appear then stop the remedy and re-asses the case. Perhaps a "proving" is in action, or perhaps the remedy has resulted in unwanted reactions. Sometimes when a symptom has been dealt with, a new one surfaces, which needs a new remedy, or perhaps the "new" symptom is a recurrence of old ones as the Law of Cure (see next chapter) runs its course.

An aggravation of symptoms indicates that the remedy is working, and provided it goes away, should be welcomed as an indication of successful treatment.

***

16. The Law of Cure in action.
***

Dr Constantine Hering formulated one of the underlying principles of homeopathy. This was The Law of Cure, which notes that during homeopathic treatment, improvement of symptoms takes place in a certain order. It begins from above and moves downwards, starting within and moving outwards, going from the major to the lesser organs and from the most recent to the earliest symptoms. The process of homeopathic treatment, as Dr Hahnemann stated, should remove the entire cause of the symptoms, and not merely suppress the symptoms.

One might consider the sequential cause approach in this matter, and treat all identified causes in the reverse of their chronological order, because that is the direction in which the Vital Force is trying to go in its efforts to heal. To consider the course of things is to consider time, and homeopathy looks at the history of the patient to determine the direction of the cure. Usually the medical history is used to understand the symptom picture and select a remedy based on symptoms, and to identify blockages to cure. However, the sequential approach treats the medical history as the very map of the disease state, and the guide to the correct remedy.

The Law of Cure was based on a lifetime's observation of the processes involved when sick patients became cured. Constantine Hering was a careful observer throughout his many years of practice and noted the order of the processes. They are expounded upon in a little more detail below.

As someone is cured, symptoms move from the innermost organs of the body (most vital to life) to the outer organs. Cure therefore moves from within to without. An example would be how someone with serious, life-threatening heart disease, can experience bowel problems during the process of cure.

Similarly, cure takes place from above to below, and symptoms fall away from the body, starting in the head, and clearing downwards, with hands or feet (or both) being affected last with skin eruptions.

Symptoms that have been suppressed in the past often resurface during the process of cure and usually do so in the reverse order of their original appearance. An example would be a patient, with heart disease, who had been successfully treated with orthodox medicines for a stomach ulcer, before the heart condition, and the appearance of stomach conditions would be welcomed as a sign that the old suppressed symptoms were being cleared out. The symptoms would be milder than the original illness. These laws apply to the treatment of chronic complaints but occasionally also to acute prescribing, so if an old symptom surfaces after a good prescribing, one should wait to see if it clears of its own accord. If it does, the remedy is still working and one should wait longer.

Suppression of a disease from the outside usually leads to a more deep-seated illness resurfacing. For example, children whose eczema has been "successfully" treated with steroids may suffer from asthma at a later date. These two events are seen by orthodox medicine as having only a casual connection, whereas the homeopath believes the suppression of the eczema has caused the asthma.

Successful homeopathic treatment involves the eczema reappearing at some point. It is also possible to suppress symptoms with doses of homeopathic medicine aimed at single symptoms only, and not taking the whole person into account.

Homeopaths use the Law of Cure to monitor treatment and to see whether the cure is going in the right direction. As far as acute or home prescribing is concerned, occasionally a well-selected constitutional remedy will push old symptoms, that may have been forgotten, to the surface. They will clear of their own accord and while they are active another remedy should not be prescribed as they might then go back in again.

It may be that any localised alteration of the state of the patient, even as small as an abscess or ulcer, is an indication that the general state is in a disturbed order. Localised imbalances can therefore be seen as barometers of what is happening inside the person, and only appear after the centre of the being has been disturbed, via the emotions, mentals, and later physicals, in the order of the Law of Cure. Every acute malady begins with general disturbance, changes of temper, character, sleep, then appetite, followed by localised disturbances in the body. Cure takes place in the same way, along the same pathways, in the same order. Palliation (suppression of symptoms) for the patient's comfort or vanity, will not cure the disturbance or fundamental cause within the patient. Surface maladies are merely the external manifestations of the inner imbalance, and need to be seen as pointers to correct remedies. A good remedy will first modify the inner problems, leading to a feeling of being better, and then will follow the pattern of the Law of Cure until at the end of the process the surface symptoms vanish. The inside needs to be put in order before the exterior symptoms are approached. The Law of Cure is the homeopath's compass and rudder in his struggle to treat the fundamental disease.

***

17. Modalities.
***

Modalities are the factors which aggravate or improve symptoms, feelings or conditions. They assist the homeopath in selecting a remedy, far quicker, by eliminating many wrong ones, and by pointing to correct ones. There are so many homeopathic remedies for each disorder, that simply looking for "PAIN" will not find the most closely matching remedy for the specific pain. The fact that the ailment hurts is not sufficient to tell the homeopath which remedy to use. But the modalities of the pain – the kind of pain it is, where the pain is, and when it hurts most – will help enormously. These are some of the factors one needs to address. For example, if the pain pulsates and burns in the leg, in addition to having certain modalities such as worse on the left side, and in the evening, and better from cold applications, then you will be able to find the most curative remedy for the leg pain. Modalities are always very important factors in choosing the most closely matching homeopathic remedy, to the totality of the simillimum. They can be the deciding factors between several remedies which may be strongly indicated. Modalities are the modifying influences and circumstances which either ameliorate (influences which make the symptoms of a condition feel better), or aggravate (influences which make the symptoms of a condition feel worse). Modalities include many factors and stimuli as perceived by the patient. Modalities may have to do with temperature, weather, climate, movement, activity, time, right and left side, sensations, physical contact, foods, drinks. They are the sensory manner and mode of how the symptoms are felt by the individual, and they are a most important criterion in choosing the right remedy.

Committing modalities to memory can aid the homeopath in prescribing remedies, although he must be sure of his facts.

There are innumerable modalities, but some frequently found ones are time of day, movement and position, and draughts. Environments are also modalities, making a patient feel better or worse, such as being at the seaside, in sunshine or shade, outside or inside, wet or dry, cold or warm, in different seasons, in warmth or cold, closed in or exposed, covered or uncovered, swaddled, standing or sitting, crouching or being in a fetal position. Rhythms should also be considered, such as repetitions, seasonal changes, at noon, and so forth.

Modalities are circumstances and conditions which affect or modify a particular symptom or state of a patient as a whole. They are aggravations or ameliorations of particular complaints or the state of the patient as a whole, with regard to various factors. Boericke alone lists several hundred modalities in his Materia Medica.

Modalities are extremely valuable to the prescribing homeopath, and rank second in importance only to the mental/emotional symptoms. Their value lies in helping to distinguish whether a remedy will work or not. For instance, one cannot expect success from a remedy which is better for heat, when the patient symptom picture is worse for heat. Modalities help to eliminate incorrect remedies quickly and help in selecting the simillimum.

***

18. Arnica, used to show how many uses each remedy can have.

***

Arnica is the most commonly used homeopathic remedy in the world, and once one has tried it for the treatment of injuries, one might consider it a miracle remedy. Its success is almost guaranteed and it should be in everyone's medicine box. Arnica, or Monk's Hood, flowers at high altitude, and is traditionally smeared on aching muscles by hikers, in high places. The dried leaves have been smoked as a kind of tobacco in various parts of the world, and its flowers, if inhaled when freshly crushed, cause sneezing and hence its name of "sneezewort". It is much more effective in homeopathic form. It is highly recommended for any kind of trauma, whether accidental or intentional. It will reduce swelling dramatically as well as relieve pain and bruising. Surgeons wonder why Arnica–taking patients did not develop the usual bruising, and do not require pain-relieving medication. The best success in Arnica is in immediate use in quite high potencies, 30C and above, although it works in lower potencies too, but then needs to be taken much more frequently in higher dose quantities. Arnica can be combined with any drug with no side-effects at all. Newborns and mothers can take Arnica to reduce the trauma of childbirth. After a sports injury it is best to take it until the injury is almost healed.

This remedy can be applied in cream form to injuries that have not broken the skin, as Arnica will irritate an open wound or cut. The cream, also known as Traumeel cream, is rubbed into sore joints and muscles to relieve discomfort. Old fisherman can rub it into their hands every day to keep them limber and less sore.

For broken bones it is often felt that nothing more can be done after splinting and pain management. However there are basic nutrients and homeopathic remedies that can reduce the pain as well as speed up the healing of the bone. Initially one should use Arnica to reduce pain and swelling, before using Symphytum (Comfrey, Knitbone) to aid healing of the bone and if there is deep bone pain, then Eupatorium may be used.

Sports people use Arnica for rapid recovery during times of heavy training, and for the quick recovery of injuries.

Head injuries may result in residual symptoms for days or even weeks or months, and Arnica can help greatly for this. Any injury to the nervous system, such as catching a finger in a car door, will benefit from Arnica, which can also be used in conjunction with various other homeopathic remedies. It is very good for relieving pain after dental work has damaged nerve-ends. Arnica will speed up healing and reduce edema and bruising after any sort of procedure where the body has been cut or traumatised.

Arnica is a highly recommended remedy for pets, especially good for bruises, and emotional or physical trauma. It is good for muscles aches and sprains, strains and injuries, as well as injuries of the brain and spinal cord, and post-operative shock. People in a lot of pain and fearful of being touched, enjoy great pain relief and calming from Arnica. Rats, dogs, budgies and horses respond well to Arnica and injured sheep naturally graze Arnica in the mountains, seeking it out. The author has used Arnica successfully for trauma, shock, depression and grief in patients.

To sum up, the main uses of Arnica are as follows:

Smelly breath.

Injury problems, mental/emotional and/or physical.

Aches and pains, bruises, sore glands.

Shock or associated problem of fears, memory.

After dentistry.

Blood blisters.

Boils, small, sore.

Broken bones with swelling.

Childbirth.

Intentional injury, surgery, sport.

Whooping coughs, bloodshot eyes, chest pains, nosebleeds.

Eye injuries.

Head injuries, lumps from knocks.

Wounds.

Joint pains, especially worse for touch.

Sprains, ankle, foot, wrist.

Strains, over-exertion.

Some toothaches.

Insomnia after over-tiredness.

Bed feels too hard.

Cannot bear to be touched, great sensitivity to pain.

Gout, rheumatism which cannot be touched.

Inflammation of different sorts.

Can be taken before OR after the event.

Jetlag, and consequent disorientation.

Heart attacks.

High fevers.

Listlessness.

Lack of energy.
Depression.
Anticipatory anxiety if expecting a fearsome experience.
Overwork and all its problems.
Haemorrhages, not too major.
Falls.
Hoarseness, especially in singers.
Aversion to touch.
Fears of death.
Taciturnity.
Nightmares, robbers, muddy water, past horror, mortal fears.
Too rapidly irritated.
Morose and morbid imaginations.
Those who refuse to see a doctor, who are ill but deny it.
Hypochondria.
Wanting to be left alone.
Feelings of helplessness, indifference, hopelessness, poor sleep.
Clutching heart with fear after nightmares.
Absentmindedness, poor concentration.
Hot head cold body.
Eczema.
Tennis elbow.
Foul smelling stools, possible faecal incontinence in sleep.
***

19. The placebo effect.
***

This phenomenon has been so well publicised over the past few decades that it needs no introduction here. Suffice it to say that a body receiving what it perceives to be a curative substance, will sometimes cure itself spontaneously, even if the substance is inert (a placebo).

Over the years, various closed-minded people, and bigots, have tried to discredit homeopathy, some saying it is merely a placebo effect that we see. In their ignorance and vitriol, they choose to disregard the millions of human adults, babies, birds, aquatic creatures, and animals which are healed or assisted across the world every single day. In the testing of homeopathic products, the people they are tested on are frequently unaware of what they are taking, thinking it is merely a sugar pill. Babies never know what they are taking, and neither do birds, animals, fish or other reptiles, yet they respond in the same way, to the same remedies.

Arnica, for instance, has the same effects on any creature anywhere in the world.

The author has no experience of using homeopathic remedies on plants but is aware that various people have tried them and had excellent results. Silica, for instance, can perk up a drooping plant.

Crocodiles, which suffer from similar medical problems to humans, such as influenza, may respond to conventional drugs in the same way as we do, and also benefit from homeopathic remedies. Of course there may be instances, as is the case with orthodox medicines, and many complementary therapies, where a placebo effect does cure

a patient, and everyone should be grateful for this happening.
***

20. Manufacture of remedies. You could make your own.
***

Hahnemann devised his system of "potentisation" which he used with spectacular effect in the preparation of his remedies. Since material doses of a remedy sometimes led to unwanted side-effects, he diluted them until the side-effects disappeared, and by succussing the diluted remedy he found that it became more potent. In fact with serial dilution and succussing, from groups of tens to hundreds and then to thousands, he increased the potency enormously while eliminating all side-effects. Dilution is usually conducted with forty percent alcohol (in some cases the alcohol content may be increased or changed according to the beliefs of the particular manufacturer) and sixty percent double distilled water mix, in a sterilized container. After three days of soaking (although this time span is varied according to who is making the remedies, and can actually be extended in extreme cases to three weeks as with Bryonia), in the case of soluble substances, the solution is strained and becomes the "mother tincture", from which a small quantity (termed one unit) is removed and again mixed with an alcohol/water solution of ninety-nine units in size, and the mix is then vigorously shaken and jolted, a process termed "succussing", and then repeated as many times as required. In the case of 1:99 units the solution has been diluted 1C (and with each successive succussing it becomes 2C, 3C etc). When it has been repeated thirty times it becomes 30C. With each process the remedy increases in potency. Hand-made remedies are very effective, although factory-made ones are now freely available. The Korsakov machine is very useful in this regard and homeopaths are divided into three camps about the most effective way to make remedies. There are those who believe only in hand-made remedies, those who believe only in machine-made ones and those who think both are fine. It can take days to make the remedies.

Excellent results are acquired with various potencies, with 30C being possibly the most popular in the UK, and was also so with Hahnemann, although Kent and the modern European homeopaths tend to use lower potencies such as 12C or 6C. In the case of insoluble in water or alcohol, substances, like Silica (Flint), the substance is ground with lactose powder in the ratio of one part flint to ninety-nine parts lactose, and then one part of the product is ground again with ninety-nine parts lactose, and then the process is repeated once more, for a third serial trituration, and then diluted and succussed in the same fashion as soluble substances. This is termed "trituration".

According to Avogadro's Law, after a 12C potency has been reached, there are no remaining molecules of the original base substance, but the medicines remain extremely effective.

Unmedicated tablets or sugar, lactose or sucrose pills are dipped into the 30C solution, which adheres to the tablet surface, and after drying, the tablets can be administered to patients requiring a 30C dose of Silica. Saturation of the pills is preferable and the process may vary a little depending on the constituency of the tablet. I have read a report about soft tablets which absorb the potentised remedy quite deeply, while other, harder tablets, are coated with the potentised remedy which stays on the surface. Pills can be purchased from various manufacturers, or can be made at home with a number of pill-making machines which are on the market, many starting with the grinding of the sugar/sucrose/lactose into fine powder before compression into a reasonably robust pillule or tablet. Tablets may be shaped differently from balls to flat to oblong ones. In my own purchases I have found that some tablets are a lot harder than other ones, for instance.

The entire process should be kept distanced from mobile telephones, microwave ovens, direct sunlight, heat, strong odours, radiation and strong magnetic fields, and of course damp and human touch.

Medicated tablets are be stored in tinted bottles of various shapes and sizes, and kept in wooden or cardboard boxes, or leather wallets or plastic boxes, all of which keep the sun or direct light off them. They should be stored in dark, dry places like drawers. Sometimes they are kept in plastic containers with tightly sealed tops.

***

21. Miasms.

***

What Hahnemann meant by the term "miasm".

***

Hahnemann referred to the possible nuclear imprint of a burned out disease, which continued to affect the Vital Force, leaving a patient prone to certain ailments and symptoms throughout life, like the ghost of the original disease. The disease itself is no longer there, only the residue. The ghost that remains is manifested in the disordered state of the internal economy, or the inside of the organism.

This residue, or ghost of the disease, is the legacy of a past chronic disease which has mistuned the living organism with small, often unnoticed beginnings. These have steadily removed the healthy state, overrunning the life force which fails to contain them, and so they have proliferated, causing more and more alteration within the living organism. They sometimes result in the death of the organism. Chronic diseases arrive from this dynamic infection of the organism, by a chronic miasm.

Miasm is derived from the Greek word "miasma", meaning taint, stain or pollution, and Hahnemann identified three primary miasms, which were the Syphilitic, Sycotic and Psoric miasms. At this point at least another seven major miasms have been identified and a further number of possible other miasms.

Chronic diseases represent those features most prevalent in their causative miasms. Miasms damage the basic functions of perpetual maintenance, growth and repair, and defence against parasites, bacteria etc. This is what allows the chronic diseases to live and grow within the organism. The symptoms of a chronic disease can point the way to identifying a miasm.   All species suffer from miasms. When a remedy does not work, or works less and less, it can be an indication that a miasm is present and that miasm needs to be treated first. A miasm will block the action of a simillimum.

Miasmic taints can also be passed on to further generations, via the nuclear imprint on proteins (a possible explanation), where miasms are inherited, but not genetically, because they can be cured.

Miasms leave a predisposition to certain ailments and symptoms, which can follow a patient for life, if not cured by anti-miasmic remedies.   These symptoms manage to elude the body's natural defences because the Vital Force has been polluted or damaged by the miasm.

At the end of the day, a miasm is nothing more than a disturbance or disruption of the normal healthy functions of the Vital Force. The miasm disrupts the normal self-healing functions of the body.

***

The miasm that Hahnemann believed to be the most common.

***

Hahnemann believed the psoric miasm was most common and it was the mother of almost all diseases.   The primary manifestation is an infectious skin eruption, that is itchy, scaly or scabby. If allowed to progress it can manifest itself in virtually innumerable symptoms, which go on to increase and torment the living organism to the end of its life. Hahnemann found that anti-psoric remedies used on psoric miasms, enabled an effective cure.

A psoric miasm within a host body can be modified by things like climate, peculiar and physical characteristics of the body it is in, mental delays, excesses and abuses, diet passions, habits and various customs. This could result in many illnesses and symptoms, treated by orthodox medicine as individual, independent phenomena, but seen by Hahnemann as all based on the same beginnings.

In order to cure a psoric miasm, (the most common miasm), a very particular and strict totality of signs must be collected, in order to prescribe a remedy for the individual and unique patient. An orthodox approach, removing surface symptoms, merely increases internal pressure, resulting in outbreaks of other symptoms. A (chronic) psoric miasm can be well hidden, requiring deep questioning even as far as ancestor history, wild delusions, dreams and apparently unrelated symptoms, to identify the remedy.

The psora goes back the farthest in history, and stems from an itch. It has been described as a monstrous, internal, chronic miasm, which is a real fundamental cause and producer of all many other forms of disease.

Psora is passed on through hundreds of generations in a bloodline and has produced an innumerable variety of defects, injuries, derangements and sufferings. Hahnemann identified three major miasms with seventy-five percent of them being psoric. However, there has been development in the field, and David Little identifies seven major worldwide miasms and a number of smaller

endemic miasms.   These may have originally been included in the psoric miasms (some of them perhaps).
***

Skin conditions and miasms.
***

Treating skin conditions with dermatological, orthodox, medicines, can cause problems. Yet skin disorders cause huge emotional distress to many people, especially females.
***

Miasms and chronic diseases are sometimes manifested by skin conditions such as jaundice, itches, eczema, herpes, dry skin, discomfort with no discharge or pus, cracks in hands and feet, profuse and/or offensive sweats, cancers, pimples, spots, acne, warts, keloids, growths, ulcers, boils and suchlike. Dermatological treatment suppresses these symptoms, which may be there for pressure release, or escape valves, for the fundamental problem which is the cause of it all.

Treating the symptoms is akin to removing the warning signals and closing the release valves, causing ever-increasing activity of the fundamental cause.   Other diseases then pop up, with different symptoms sometimes, and in different parts of the host body. Psora may also develop immunity to the medicines being used on the surface, resulting in less and less success in symptom removal.   Symptoms in any event, according to Hahnemann, will recur perhaps year after year, and their treatment will not in any way cure the deep-seated cause. In epidemics, treatments of surface symptoms to suppress them, has resulted in all conditions being magnified and intensified.

It is far better to treat the miasm, which will result in the disappearance of dermatological symptoms, than it is to suppress the symptoms and leave the miasm intact, which will cause it to produce more complicated and more serious problems, not necessarily skin-related either. An example of this might be that removal of warts (an external manifestation of a miasm), can result in asthma, an internal manifestation of a miasm, appearing.

It is useless to remove only one part or another of the syndrome. The remedy must be similar to all the manifesting symptoms, the background and the underlying cause. The simillimum must reflect the constitutional factors, the causation, and the totality of signs and symptoms. This is the basis of Hahnemann's miasmic doctrine.

There can also be more than one miasm present. Skin problems are only one single indicator of a possible miasm. On the same principle, Kent comments that the symptoms of asthma can never be cured unless the underlying miasm is addressed.

A miasm may destroy, or severely curtail sporting activities.
***

Anti-psoric (psoric miasm) remedies.
***

An anti-psoric remedy should be given once only, initially in high potency. Some sources say 30C and others 200C). An aggravation of symptoms (healing crisis) may come and go but nothing more should be given until its effect has worn off. This may take anything from days to months and in extreme cases perhaps years. The psora may have been in existence for years or even generations and cannot be cured overnight. Some examples of allopathic names for psoric symptoms are convulsions, mania, imbecility, madness, epilepsy, scoliosis, cancer, gout, haemorrhage from nose, lungs, bladder, asthma, impotence, deafness, urinary calculus, defects of the senses, and numerous types of pains. This is the tip of the iceberg only. The psora is clearly deep seated, firmly ensconced and powerful enough to kill the hosting body. The anti-psoric remedy needs time to work effectively in activating and strengthening the Vital Force sufficiently for it to recognise and deal with the miasm and all its symptoms. The Vital Force needs some time to do its job properly and restore health and balance.

There are further problems which may arise if anti-psoric remedies are given too frequently. These are that either the body may reflect the dosage, rendering it of no value, or alternatively symptoms could arise which in themselves could need further treatment. These are the inappropriate or counter-productive effects of too strong and prolonged a dose. Some of the conditions which could manifest are things such as acidity, burning, cancers, carcinomas, constipation, epilepsy, flatulence, hoarseness, itching of the skin, leprosy, burning of the spinal cord, watery discharge from nose and eyes, with burning. There are also highs and lows, struggling with the outside world, lack of confidence, anxiety, fears, inability to cope, insecurity, but always mentally alert, with hope, to name some of them.

The psoric miasm is a disturbance in cellular homeostasis (equilibrium), making cells prone to infection and inflammation, with functional abnormalities occurring (e.g. hormone problems). The skin is usually the first to react, followed by progress into deeper, more vital organs. Bowels and lungs can be affected, resulting in inflammatory bowel disorders or bronchitis. Overproduction of cells can also result, with warts, tumours and spondylosis (spinal degeneration) occurring. Incorrect dosage could result in some of these symptoms not being addressed properly.

Miasms have mysterious and persistent progressions and only very experienced homeopaths should attempt to treat them. Hahnemann was aware of the Third Book of Moses in the Bible, (Leviticus) where the word "psora" is mentioned, referring to a proneness to disruptive diseases. Psora have been known for a long time.

Sometimes an anti-psoric remedy may work partially and many more symptoms may arise, from another previously hidden miasm or disease. These might need to be treated first before the original miasm can be treated again. Diseases and miasms can be layered, so a new assessment may need to be made after the effect of the first, single, anti-psoric remedy has been noted and observed. A series of different, possibly related remedies, may be required to remove miasmic layers. A prior knowledge of the order in which these layers have arrived, will help greatly.

This is why these remedies should be given once only, until their effect has worn off, and to see whether they are appropriate in a second or further application.

One comment which I read, was that giving too deep an acting remedy, in too large an amount, in too high a potency for the stage of the disease, results in the breaking down of the walls surrounding the bacteria, and setting it free. This related to tuberculosis and is perhaps why too much of a remedy, as mentioned above, can precipitate many of the symptoms of the remedy, or disease one is treating.

***

Psoric and syphilitic miasms.

***

The most significant pathological (medical) differences between a psoric miasm and a syphilitic miasm.

***

The psoric miasm is due to some sort of suppressed itch or skin problem, while the syphilitic miasm is thought to be an inherited problem caused by syphilitic infections in past generations. The former tends to produce irritation, inflammation and hypersensitivity, with little actual tissue degeneration, while the latter tends towards granulation, degeneration and ulceration.

Physically the psora tends to make the organism toxic, the skin unhealthy, and perverts the functions of the digestive and eliminative organs. Syphilis tends to cause congenital defects, asymmetrical bony structure, deformed teeth and the classic forward-protruding lower jaw some creatures, especially human beings.

The psora is expressive and noisy, and full of self-deception. Sufferers may seem foolish and impractical. Syphilis has some madness and some genius and some irony and obsession with destruction. Sufferers can feel self-destructive (cutting skin for instance), and end in idiocy or insanity.

Psoric miasms result in itchy, crawling, tickling and burning pains (periodic sometimes or alternating with a congested chest), which are absent in syphilitic miasms.

Psora has scanty, irritating and itchy discharges, while syphilis has offensive, foul, putrid, smelly discharges.

Psoric skin is dry, rough, unhealthy, with little injuries becoming infected and itchy. Syphilis has brownish red or coppery coloured spots, eruptions that do not itch, and a tendency towards ulceration.

These then are the fundamental and significant pathological differences between the psoric and syphilitic miasms. However there are more, noteworthy and significant factors which highlight the differences.

Psora has restlessness and despair, dread and a tendency to forget, while syphilis has depression and self-destruction, either conscious or unconscious (see self-abuse).

Psora has a tendency to parasitic infection, like worms and fungus, which are absent in syphilis.

Syphilis has bony outgrowths and bony bumps (spine etc) which are absent in psora.

Psora is both hungry and better after rest, while syphilis is not hungry and is not better after rest.

Syphilis likes being in water, while psora dislikes it.

Syphilis has weak ligaments, with a tendency to sprains and strains, which psora does not have.

Syphilis is forgetful and loses ideas, has lymphatic and glandular problems, bloody discharges, irregular teeth and poor hygiene, of which none is common to psora.

Syphilis is better for mountains.

It is difficult for me to highlight the most significant difference between the two, as there are so many significant differences. However, I would suggest that a very significant pathological difference is the proneness to tissue degeneration in syphilis, which is absent in psora. Syphilitic conditions involve destructive processes like skin ulcers, many neuromuscular diseases, and stomach ulcers, while psora produces inflammations and functional disturbances, such as dermatitis, cystitis, bronchitis, and some types of anaemia.

***

22. The Bach flower remedies.
***

No study of homeopathy can be complete unless it includes a good look at Dr Edward Bach's remedies. Without the emotional system, and mood, in good order, it can be very difficult to function effectively in the arena of life.

Bach remedies are based on personality, and so whatever the problem might be, the homeopath should select the remedy according to emotional outlook, mood, temperament and personality.

When considering Bach remedies, one focuses on the emotional and mental symptoms of the patient. These symptoms are also essential in seeking a constitutional remedy, and Bach knew that the emotional and mental symptoms should be the mainstay of ones treatment of any chronic condition. Bach's main contribution was his focus on the outlook and life of the distressed patient, rather than only the disease symptoms (physical). This was a considerable breakthrough for a physician and bacteriologist of the 1930's. He realized that disequilibrium of the mind was a prime cause of all ailments.

Using Bach as a basis, one can focus on any negative mental states which are preventing the body from healing itself. Bach found that we can classify people into groups by the way they eat, talk, use body language and move, and thereby display their mental states. Giving up his practice, he investigated the situation further, so paving the way for homeopaths of the future to be able to recognise and cure negative states, which prevented cure. When using Bach Flower Remedies we focus on the details of the patient's mental state, and change the state by administering the appropriate Flower Remedies. Once happiness is restored, in the form of inner harmony, the person thinks clearly, does the appropriate things to cure himself, effects internal cure by using the Vital Force, and throws off the mood which had brought him down. If not treated soon enough, bad attitudes and moods can snowball into major states of unbearable anguish and ill-health.

We know that when a system is out of balance or mistuned, a negative state creeps in, which can be associated with either personality, or be a transient mental state created by the circumstances and conditions of life. Look at job change, bereavement, disappointment, isolation, infirmity, losses, unpleasant environments, and you find anxiety, anger, depression, impatience, unhappiness, and these alter our well-being and we feel ill and look older. Edward Bach knew this and treated the negative outlooks with flower remedies. We follow suit and look for negative outlooks when considering flower remedies.

Bach identified 7 basic groupings for us to consider. Each group headed the emotional states curable under that heading. He developed 38 remedies to cure these negative states. We need to focus on each heading, and then its subsections, when considering the flower remedies. They are, briefly:

Fear – terror, panic, fears, shyness, of anger, the unknown etc.

Uncertainty – judgement, need others, moods, dejected, despair, fatigue, indecision.

Lack of interest – dream, escape, past, apathy, drifting, thoughts in a circle, gloom.

Loneliness – quiet, intelligent, impatient, intolerant, self-interested.

Over-sensitive to influence and ideas – inner torture, weak, habits, hate, jealousies.

Despondency and despair – expect failure, blame self, overwhelmed, shock, self-pity.

Over-care for welfare of others – possessive, nagging, perfectionist, insensitivity, ruthless, leaders, overworkers.

***

By focussing on the above we can select a Flower Remedy. There are also remedies available for no less than 6 sleep disorders, including unwanted thoughts, and also a Rescue Remedy for all traumas and shocks.

When considering Bach remedies, we need to remember that good health is harmony, rhythm, positivity, constructivity and general happiness. Ill-health is negativity, unhappiness and destructive attitude. The entry of Bach, into the world of emotions in diagnosing health, started when he found that fear caused asthma in a patent. On this he developed his life work.

***

Rescue Remedy, its constituents and what each component is useful for.

Rescue Remedy may be taken internally (pillules or drops) or applied externally (cream or liquid or sprays) to stings, strains, bruises etc. It alleviates mental anguish, so enabling the body to start the healing process without delay. Animals which have suffered from any shock or terror can also benefit from this remedy. Even plants respond well to a few drops of the remedy. Bach selected the 5 elements of Rescue Remedy because he felt they combine to form an effective all-round crisis remedy, as he first demonstrated with shipwrecked sailors, who recovered amazingly after being dosed with it.

The uses of each component are listed below, and then expounded upon, quite briefly. Together they form a mode of treatment for almost any sort of trauma.

Impatiens: Tension and stress.

Star of Bethlehem: Shock.

Cherry Plum: Desperation.

Rock Rose: Terror.

Clematis: Feeling faint.

Impatiens, as the name suggests, is useful for treating irritability, nervousness, impatience, frustration, rush, impetuosity, and mental tension associated with those who want everything done their own way fast. It encourages less haste, relaxation, tolerance, gentleness and acceptance of others. Patients learn to wait and become less fretful and jumpy and stop fidgeting. They regain their poise.

Star of Bethlehem is indicated wherever there is shock, disturbing news, distressing sights, bereavement, pain and sorrow, sometimes stemming back to events of years before. It can neutralize sudden or delayed shocks and sadness, and is a welcome comforter and soother. Fright and disappointment can also be treated with this remedy.

Cherry Plum is indicated in treating patients who feel their minds are giving way. It is for the desperate fear of losing mental control and sanity, and doing the self harm. It is indicated for those with thoughts of suicide. Sometimes there can be sudden murderous and violent impulses with complete loss of control in some instances. *Cherry Plum* can restore calm, quiet courage, and the ability to survive and endure the knocks of life.

Rock Rose is the treatment for extreme fear, terror and panic. It may not be rational but is still very real. It may be caused from mimicking others, near escapes, seeing an accident, nightmares, television or radio broadcasts, approaching tornadoes etc. The terror may prevent normal behaviour patterns such as a person not being able to go to sleep because of the terror of nightmares. It is good to note that ***Rock Rose*** is indicated for fear which creates terror and panic, and not simply for known fears when ***Mimulus*** would be indicated. It restores courage, strength of will and character, and the ability to care for others first.

Clematis is indicated for a feeling of faintness, lack of interest in the present, vacant look, inattentiveness, obliviousness to surroundings, boredom, lack of concentration, loss of the thread of a conversation, mental escapism and living in a dreamlike state. There is absentmindedness, sleepiness, listlessness, withdrawal and dreaming. Things are too slow for Clematis. The remedy inspires lively interest, action, mastery over thoughts and activities, and realistic down to earth activity.
***

Bach remedies.
Inner torture with brave exterior put forward, ***Agrimony.***
Unfounded fears, ***Aspen.***
Intolerance, ***Beech.***
Timid and weak-willed, ***Centaury.***
Doubts self, must asks others for advice, ***Cerato.***
Fears insanity, wants to shout for help, ***Cherry Plum.***
Continues to make same mistakes, ***Chestnut bud.***

Over-possessive and selfish, **Chicory.**
Dreamers, vacant minds, **Clematis.**
Self-hatred, disgust, feels unclean internally and externally, **Crab Apple.**
Overwhelmed by responsibility, **Elm.**
Melancholy, discouraged, despondent, **Gentian.**
Hopeless, no hope nor faith, **Gorse.**
Obsessed with own ailments and trivia, **Heather.**
Aggression, suspicion, envy, hatred, jealousy, **Holly.**
Nostalgic, anchored in the past, **Honeysuckle.**
Cannot cope, mental fatigue, fears the day, **Hornbeam.**
Irritable, impatient, frustrated, **Impatiens.**
Certain of failure, feels inferior, zero confidence, **Larch.**
Fear of normal things, secret fears, **Mimulus.**
Sudden bouts of severe gloom, despair, **Mustard.**
Needs relentless effort to continue, desperate but fights on, **Oak.**
Vitality totally gone, exhausted, **Olive.**
Always feels guilty, blames self, **Pine.**
Mother hen always panicking about others, expects the worst, **Red Chestnut.**
Completely rigid mind, a martyr, self-denial, seeks own perfection, over-religious, **Rock Water.**
Cannot choose, indecision, opposite moods alternately afflict patient, **Scleranthus.**
Disappointment, bad news, shock, fright, **Star of Bethlehem.**
Terrible mental despair and suffering, anguish, loneliness, only blackness ahead, **Sweet Chestnut.**
Will overwhelms physical strength, fanatical, perfectionism, tackles too much, **Vervain.**

Expects total obedience, no grasp that others have feelings, craves authority, a tyrant, *Vine.*

Stuck with fixed attachments to the past, cannot go ahead, may be a person, a bad habit, cannot throw off reverence to fixed ideas, *Walnut.*

Condescending, aloof, disdainful, completely rigid, *Water Violet.*

Mental arguments about past events, persistent repetition, troubled and angry, pre-occupied, *White Chestnut.*

Uncertain, undecided, cannot choose life path, keeps trying things to match talents but frustration results, talented and ambitious, very bored, *Wild Oat.*

Resignation, apathy, gives up, expressionless, *Wild Rose.*

Bitterness, self-pity, resentment, blames everyone else, *Willow.*

***

23. Tissue salts, essential for full health. Emotional disorders often follow ill-health.
***

Included in the huge range of homeopathic remedies, are twelve inorganic tissue salts. Bodies have a critical need for each of these to be present in the correct balance and quantity, in order for them to be free of disease and pain. Below is a list of them all, their functions, and what occurs when there is a deficiency or imbalance. You should eat plenty of fresh vegetables and fruit in your balanced diet. The remedies listed below, are listed with the conditions they may cure, and these conditions occur when the salt by the same name as the remedy, is in short supply. Eat healthily!
***

Calc fluor: Glandular tumours, venous problems, prolapses, bone problems. This salt is an essential component of bone surfaces, elastic fibres and tooth enamel. When elasticity is gone, then serious problems can ensue. These include the dilation of blood vessels, tumours, piles, enlarged veins, heart enlargement, relaxed (flabby) inner organs and prolapses.
***

Calc phos: Anaemia, bloat, bone problems, development of the body, teeth. A shortage of this salt results in bone disease, and bones remain weak and undeveloped if deprived of it in the developmental stages. It plays a major part in the digestion and absorption of nutrients. Absence or shortage of it may produce anaemia, spasms, convulsions and rotting teeth. It is essential for recovery from wasting diseases, and restores a shortage of red corpuscles. Young creatures deprived of this salt, display emaciation, suppuration of bones, and spinal weakness. Later on, fractures will not heal, rheumatism may appear, and certain glands may enlarge significantly. Faeces may be hot and disgusting, with a generally sick stomach and vomitting.

***

Calc sulph: Catarrh, boils, suppuration, carbuncles. A shortage results in various abscesses. An excellent remedy for all ailments where pus-formation is liable, or has already developed. It is good for lung diseases, with heavy, yellow pus anywhere in or on the body.

***

Ferr phos: Congestion, inflammation, fevers. A good remedy for early stage congestion, inflammation and fevers, since it attracts oxygen and assists oxygen transportation in the blood. It strengthens the walls of blood vessels and supplies the red colour in blood corpuscles. It is excellent for anaemia, pneumonia, inflamed rheumatism, nosebleeds, incontinence and apoplexies. Symptoms are aggravated by motion.

***

Kali mur: A second stage remedy for inflammatory diseases, croup, catarrh, pneumonia, swollen glands, eustachian deafness and diarrhoea. It is good for all inflammations and exudations, and should follow Ferr phos. Second stage symptoms involve thick, white expectorations with a white or grey covering of the tongue. There may also be skin eruptions with yellow-pus pimples, ulcers and rheumatic swellings. Car-sickness is common.

***

Kali phos: Brain, nerves, muscles, blood vessels. Supplies the brain's nerve fluid. This salt is a good remedy for sleeplessness and nervous conditions, and any nerve degeneracy (neurasthenia). Some examples would be, no nerve power, prostration, mental exhaustion, brain-fag, forms of insanity, forms of paralysis, epilepsy, hysteria, no co-ordination of extremities, and blood decomposition. Examples include haemorrhages, gangrene, carrion-smelling diarrhoea, typhoid, incontinence, itches, dizziness, breathing problems, wheezing, headaches and a dark yellow tongue. The patient cannot stand noise or physical activity.
***

Kali sulph: Third stage of inflammatory or catarrhal condition, diarrhoea, skin diseases, rheumatism, ulcerations and flatulence. The salt carries oxygen, which is a body's primary source of fuel, so therefore it is the fountain of all vitality. It assists with yellowish, watery secretions with a slimy, yellow tongue, and is good for inflamed throats, coughs, pneumonia, skin diseases with yellow pus, diarrhoea and eye problems. It may be used for scurfy or scaly skins and various ailments, which are much worse when the patient is warm.
***

Mag phos: Spasms, cramps, convulsions, epilepsy. This salt is a constituent of muscle, nerves, brain, bone, spine, teeth and blood corpuscles. Shortage of the salt causes spasms and convulsions, and is related to nerve cells and muscle tissue. It can help in tetanic contractions, twitches and jerks, fits, coughs, paralysis and retention of urine. It is used for pains in the head, face, teeth, stomach, heart and

limbs, and has been described as the "homeopathic aspirin". Sometimes there is prostration with an extremely tympanic abdomen, with flatus. There may be dysentry. Pains may move around and are sudden and piercing. Massage and warmth may help.
***

Nat mur: Catarrh with watery secretions, as in skin disease, constipation, diarrhoea, hay fever, colds and influenza. This salt regulates the volume of water in each cell of the body. It is found in every single cell of the entire body, both in liquids and in solids. Distribution of water within a system, if not as it should be, can cause dryness in some places and too much wetness in others. Mucus membranes react violently to this. Dis-equilibrium may also occur in the lymphatic system, blood, spleen, liver and stomach linings. Non-optimal distribution causes headaches, stomach aches, general aches and problems with secretions like tears, mucus or water, which can be too little or too much. This remedy can help with wet mucus-froth from skin eruptions, watery blisters with crusts and various other skin problems. Constipation or very wet eyes can sometimes be treated with this salt, as can eye infections, slimy bubble-covered tongues and coryza from anywhere. Other diseases of the pharynx, bladder, chest and some glands can also be cured.
***

Nat phos: Intestines, diarrhoea, worms and sour-acid vomitting. This salt assists in the elimination of both excess sugar and lactic acid. The latter can be a residue of physical overstress, and leave stiffness and pain. The remedy also reduces sour acid belching, fermentation,

vomitting and green, stinking diarrhoea, with colic and spasms caused by mouth acid. The tongue is wet-yellow, with yellow discharge, a sure sign indicating this remedy. The eyes may release yellow pus. The bladder function may be affected and worms may take hold in the gut. Rheumatic pains often accompany these symptoms, together with itches, skin problems, crusts and pain.
***

Nat sulph: Liver, nausea, diarrhoea, asthma, edemas and breathing problems. This salt eliminates all extra water from the blood and regulates bile. The tongue is dark brown-green or grey-green and stools are dark green and full of excess bile from the liver. Vomitting occurs. The remedy helps with fevers, vomitting and bilious diseases. The liver is enlarged with skin eruptions and blotches. Urine may have sediment in it and skin diseases may be visible, including edemas, warts, gout-like problems, moist, yellow scales and inflammations, worse towards the front and head of the body.
***

Silica: Uterine disorders, indurations, swollen glands, carbuncles, ulceration and suppuration, foreign bodies stuck under the skin (splinters, thorns, quills). Silica is critical for all functions of the body and is only less prolific than water, in bodies. This salt acts on bones, joints, glands, skin and mucus membranes. A shortage of it results in signs of malnutrition and is excellent for undernourished patients. All ulcerations and suppurations benefit from it, as do all tendons, the periosteum and the bones. Both hardness and induration can be treated with this salt, which ripens suppurations, resulting in the escape

of pus. Hard, swollen glands may ripen, and drain. Constipation may be present. The eyes may be stye-infected and epileptic fits may occur, especially with moon changes. There can be flatulence and serious lung infections, with all the symptoms much worse at night. Full moon can precipitate various symptom attacks.
***

24. Amino acids are essential for emotional and physical health.
***

Various disorders and apparent diseases may be treated for years, but they may be caused by improper diet or incomplete digestion, with possible deficiencies in the diet. The result could be shortages or imbalances of amino acids, tissue salts, vitamins or minerals, leading to the disorders. So it is good to ensure that diet is complete before trying to treat disorders.

Amino acids are the building blocks of the body, essential to its maintenance. They build cells, repair tissues, form anti-bodies to combat bacteria and viruses, are part of the enzyme and hormonal system, build nucleoproteins (RNA, DNA), carry oxygen, and are needed for muscle activity. Eight are essential and the others can be manufactured by the body provided it is properly fed. Their absence can result in many disorders which can be mistaken for disease or infection. In the list below you can get an idea of their importance. They are acquired when the body digests protein, which it breaks down into 22 known amino acids, hence the importance of adequate protein intake.

The author has enjoyed a greatly increased physical capacity from using Branch Chain Amino Acids, as a supplement both prior to and after heavy exercise.

Essential amino acids:

Tryptophan, a natural relaxant, induces normal sleep patterns, combats anxiety, diminishes depression, reduces migraines, boosts the immune system, combats heart and artery spasms, reduces cholestrol in conjunction with *Lysine*.

Lysine, ensures absorption of calcium, helps make up bone, cartilage and connective tissues, assists production of antibodies, hormones and enzymes, may help reduce viral growth, combat herpes, and any deficiency causes anaemia, reduction in sterility, hair-loss, stunted growth, red eyes, irritation, exhaustion and poor concentration.

Methionine, supplies sulphur for hair, skin and nails, increases lecithin production and reduces cholestrol, reduces liver fat and protects kidneys, clears heavy metal accumulation, creates ammonia-free urine and reduces bladder irritation, improves hair.

Phenylalaine, used to produce norpinephrine to transmit signals from the brain to the nerve cells and back, also an anti-depressant, hunger-reducer, alert-maker and memory improver.

Threonine, helps stop fat build-up in the liver, assists digestion and keeps the intestines healthy, a constituent of tooth enamel and collagen.

Valine, calms the emotions, promotes mental vigour and muscle co-ordination.

Leucine and isoleucine, assist manufacture of biochemical components of the body, used for alertness, energy and general stimulation.

Non-essential amino acids, very briefly.

Arginine, essential for the immune system, wound healing, regeneration of liver, growth hormones for muscles.

Tyrosine, transmits nerve impulses to the brain, fights depression, assists memory, makes one alert and healthy by acting on the thyroid, adrenal and pituitary glands.

Glycine, triggers oxygen release for cell making, critical for hormone production.

Serine, stores glucose in liver and muscles, provides ant-bodies, synthesises fatty-acid sheath round nerve fibres.

Glutamic acid, brain food for improving mental capacities, healing ulcers, lifts fatigue, helps control alcoholism, schizophrenia and sugar craving.

Aspartic acid, helps expel highly poisonous ammonia, may improve endurance.

Taurine, calms possible seizures, clears free radicals.

Cystine, anti-oxidant, protects against radiation and pollution, slows ageing, assist protein digestion, needed in hair and skin.

Histidine, a component of haemoglobin, used for treating arthritis, allergies, ulcers, anaemia and poor hearing.

Proline, for joints and tendons, also keeps heart muscle strong.

Alanine, provides energy for muscle tissue, brain and nerves, produces anti-bodies, helps metabolise sugars and organic acids.

***

25. Comment on the arrangement of information.
***

Success in many of life's activities, requires continuity. The more that emotional, and mental focus and functioning, are interrupted, the more achievements diminish in number and magnitude. The purpose of this book is to limit psychological disorders, to the absolute minimum, while curing as many as possible which may make an appearance. This will result in more people making greater achievements, having more optimism, and enjoying many more years of health and success. Negative attitudes which impede function, as well as mental obstructions, can often be removed. Physical disorders can also be tended to so as to remove concomitant psychological setbacks.

All headings will appear in alphabetical order, with suggestions for treatment.

Please note that emotional and mental factors are lumped together without distinction, and also take note that there is plenty of overlap between different conditions and headings, so if you do not find the disorder you seek under one heading, then please peruse associated headings.
***

26. Bad habits leading to psychological problems.
***

Alcoholism.
Caffeine addiction.
Coffee.
Drunkenness.
Liars.
Malcontent.
Negative perspective (see below).
Smoking.
***

27. Negative perspectives.

***

A negative person sees only the negative aspects of anything at all. This becomes a habit and condition of mind. Positive interpretations of events or matters are filtered out, in favour of negative ones. Counselling and medication are usually needed to rectify the situation. Backup is also required from trained or positive people.

If treatment is not forthcoming, or the patient is unable to cure himself, then serious illness or even death might result. Suicide may be the only option contemplated, and the sufferer's quality of life may become very poor, irrespective of what they really have.

Life activities are severely reduced in effectiveness when a negative attitude pervades one's thinking. *Lach, Lyco, Staph.*

Willow (Bach).

***

28. Self-hypnosis is excellent for achieving excellence, but needs a peaceful mind.
***

Self-hypnosis can change attitudes, which in turn change behaviour, which can lead to the achievement of what may have previously seemed not possible. You can program your own mind to take instructions which it might have balked at previously.

Old, unproductive behaviour patterns, can be shed in favour of positive and productive ones. Ideas which would have previously been turned away, can now be accepted, and acted upon. Fears and phobias can be put aside, and be replaced with confidence. Concentration can be improved, and love of life can be increased.

Life can become easier and far more productive, and a winning "killer-instinct" can be fostered to replace a softer or weaker approach.

A weak ego which has led to mediocre performances in the past, can be bolstered with self-hypnosis, to become a strong ego, capable of driving one on to new heights.

There are many excellent books from which to learn, or psychologists and life-coaches who can assist one.
***

29. Neural pathways prefer peace and focus in their development.

***

When you complete an activity once, you acquire a memory of it. Each time after that, you increase the depth and effectiveness of that memory. Initially you have to think about what to do, consciously. The more you do the activity, the easier it becomes, and the less you need to consciously think about what you are doing. Finally, you can do it automatically, with no conscious thought. This happens when the neural pathway is complete, and unobstructed.

Once you no longer need a conscious thrust to activate yourself into the activity, you can do it very much faster, and more effectively, than before. You do it on automatic pilot.

A neural pathway can be likened to a path through the bush. You start by making a short inroad, cleaning some bush. Each time you clear a little more and go a little further. Finally you can walk the pathway with no obstruction. But leave it untended and unwalked for a while and the bush starts growing back, and needs to be re-cut. A neural pathway is the same. Do the activity regularly and the way is unobstructed. One can keep other matters in mind while executing the moves, such as reading a rugby field while catching a ball, and deciding which way to go. If one consciously focussed only on catching the ball, one could not read the field at the same time. Similarly, if one focussed on one's finger while playing the piano, one could not focus on the melody. The fingers need to be activated by a clear neural pathway.

A neural pathway functions perfectly when the mind is uncluttered, unobstructed by distracting thoughts and emotions. You can use this book to try reach a point of complete emotional and mental clarity.

***

30. Visualisations require a calm mind and uncluttered mental processes.

***

A great deal of achievement or good performance, is arrived at via the art of visualisation. If you have done something in your mind, over and over, you have a far better chance of doing it physically. If you are not certain what you are supposed to be doing, and have not done it in your mind, then the body will not really know what is being asked of it. Visualising can allay anxiety and worry. Visualisation applies to many walks of life, for instance, the public speaker who visualises himself making a wonderful speech, over and over, will easily achieve this without excessive fear. He will simply know in advance what is going to happen, and it will happen.

In order to visualise adequately, a completely clear mind with calm emotions is needed, as are basic visualisation techniques. You will need to achieve the correct frame of mind.

The three most effective visualisations the author uses in teaching martial arts, are, firstly, imagining being in one's own body and doing the thing. Secondly, imagine watching oneself from a camera on one's own head, as if one were a figure on a television set. Thirdly, doing the activity inside ones own head, but being aware of all factors involved, such as the sounds, the smells, the light, the people, the feeling of the ground or mat, the feel of the kit, the sensations of the activity. The same principles can be applied to almost any other activity. Homeopathy can be utilised to help achieve the correct frame of mind to do this.

Combining all these factors will give you an enormous headstart over those who do not enjoy this advantage.
***

31. Age is surrounded by misconceptions.
***

Performance declines because of different factors, frequently and erroneously attributed to age. Some of these are the numerous chronic diseases affecting people, and manifesting themselves in numerous different symptoms, which the sufferer does not see as all being part of a fundamental disease, often curable. Then there are the miasms, steadily eroding physical and mental ability, but often curable with homeopathy.

Lifestyle also plays a large part, with poor eating and sleeping habits, and stress, breaking down the mind and body's ability to perform optimally. Bad habits contribute their share to decline, being such activities as smoking, over-consumption of alcohol and caffeine.

Poor exercise schedules also diminish abilities, and the Sunday golfer, or once a week social aerobics class sportsperson, should not expect to improve with age, or even maintain what is already there. The same principle applies to the use of the brain and the exercise of correct attitudes and thoughts, all necessary to mental and emotional good health. The psychology of good habits and practices needs daily practice.

In the experience of the author, physical and mental prowess can improve steadily for decades, with proper Homeopathic treatment, unstressed practice methods, good diets, a quiet mind, correct meditation, proper diagnosis and treatment of diseases and injuries, and all the other factors which see many people into excellent performance, sometimes into their eighties. There is no reason at all to imagine that age will automatically interrupt life activities.

Interruption comes from incorrect preconceptions, and frequently (Homeopathically) curable disorders.

There is debate among interested parties, worldwide, as to how long humans are programmed to live healthy productive lives for. How long should you be able to function actively and energetically, with enjoyment, before age overtakes you? Some opinions indicate that 100 years is the genetic program, and given healthy environments we can all expect to live to that age. The author saw a 120 year old woman in Thailand, who had functioned well until a few years earlier. She could still speak and laugh and was mentally sharp.

As for scaling down one's activities, that in itself will lead to decline in performance. There are many over-sixty athletes who enjoy a daily two hour workout, whether it is climbing a mountain, going to a gym, or doing martial arts, and they annihilate younger aspiring athletes. Some martial artists do forms or kata very actively into their eighties. One karateist, at eighty, still has a most devastating punch, which knocks big, younger men flying when they hold the punchbag. Another, at 80, still teaches actively for 3 days at a time, all day long. He has just established a new international organisation to unite like-minded people.

***

32. Mental and Emotional State of Mind. (Anon).
***

If you think you are beaten, you are.

If you think you dare not, you don't.

If you'd like to win, but think you can't, you will not win.

If you think you'll lose, you've lost.

For out in the world, we find success begins with a person's will.

It's all in the state of mind.

If you think you are outclassed, you are.

You've got to think high to rise.

You've got to be sure of yourself before you can win a prize.

Life's battles and successes don't go to the stronger or faster man.

The person who succeeds is the person who thinks he can.
***

33. Treatment.

***

Where more than one possibility is listed, then you can either try the different remedies, or preferably acquire a Materia Media and see which of the suggested remedies matches the patient's picture in the most number of symptoms. Dr Bach's Flower Remedies are usually followed by (Bach). A good Materia Medica will also make other suggestions, which may be of use.

***

34. Emotional/Mental Disorders and Remedies.
***

The author suspects that possibly all ability to cope with life's challenges may relate in some way to mental and emotional factors. Every person hoping to advance and succeed in life, is encouraged to examine and heal any disorders relating to state-of-mind, as soon as possible.
***

Lack of mental clarity, peace and focus, may obstruct coping and achievement in various degrees, up to causing complete failure to achieve, or perhaps continue, with the tasks of life.
***

A.
***

Abandoned.
Thinks he will be abandoned, fears rejection, afraid of loneliness ahead.
Mimulus (Bach).
***

Ability.
Feels she has insufficient ability to handle what is ahead.
Larch, Elm (both Bach).
***

Abnormal, obsessed with own perceived strangeness.
Shame, feels dirty, full of shortcomings, flawed, unwholesome.
Crab apple (Bach).
***

Abrasiveness.

Intolerant of others, critical, irritable, superior attitude, racial, elitist, rigid in body and mind, closed-minded.
Beech, Hickory (both Bach).
***

Absenteeism, avoiding confrontation.
Wants balance and joy, hates adverse matters, hates disharmony, represses opinions to maintain peace, liver problems, no aggressive power, loves harmony and peace.
Agrimony (Bach).
***

Abstract, unreal fantasies.
Tired with fixed ideas, heavy, minimal interest in present circumstances, closed-minded, stuck, cannot adjust or adapt.
Clematis (Bach).
***

Abula (Ebula) (unable to do anything).
No reaction, unable to do anything, seemingly switched off, active life not possible.
Baryta carb, Opium, Aeth.
***

Affection, for friends and family gone.
Depression, irritability, no more interest in favourite things, finds no enthusiasm for normal duties, cannot take obligations.
Sepia.
***

Aggression.
Bell, Nux vom, Sulph.

Desperate to be the centre of attention, quarrelsome, interruptive of activities, argues, contradicts everyone, unpopularity makes him worse. *Merc sol.*
Deeply angry, cannot settle to normal living, throws things, very childish, peevish, unable to behave in adult fashion. *Staph.*
Demanding, rude, a disastrous team player, a bear with a sore head, un-cooperative, cannot read others at all, wants his own way at all times. *Nux vom.*
***

Agoraphobia.
Fears people, fears crowds, panic in gym, trains, aeroplanes, in open spaces like fields sometimes, public places, cannot get to classes because of this, misses competitions or activities with groups.
Arg nit, Lyco.
***

Ailing, constantly.
Always imagines she is ill, hypochondria, obsessed by trivialities and little problems, constantly tells everyone, exaggerates problems right out of context, no interest at all in other people.
Heather (Bach).
***

Alienated.
Not able to identify with the preconceptions of other people around. Perhaps more/less educated, foreign, from a different milieu. Often more evolved, more spiritual, more refined, self-contained, has no real need for others. Loyal, expects others to keep up with him, rigid with skin and arthritic tendencies. May fight back at those who have

alienated him, join terrorist groups, seek their destruction. Us and them attitudes, good and evil perceptions.
Water violet (Bach).
***

Alone, wants solitude and quiet, expects to be cared for, selfish.
Sepia.
Alone, shuns company, does not want to be talked to, wants due respect, grandiose dreams.
Ham.
***

Alone, fearful.
Cannot be left alone, fears death, anxious, restless, needs emotional support, needs someone else around. Derives confidence from others and cannot act alone.
Ars alb.
***

Aloof.
Disdainful, condescending, proud, rigid in mind, physically stiff.
Water violet (Bach).
***

Ambition, none.
Cannot get ahead because there is no ambition to drive improvement.
Wild rose, Gorse (both Bach).
***

Ambition thwarted, at crossroads.
Dissatisfied and ambitious but uncertain as to which path to follow. Sees various possibilities, would like guidance

which is not forthcoming, no-one to bounce ideas off. Needs life-coaching. *Wild oat (Bach).*
***

Amorous frenzy.
Fears, rages, barking and biting, lewd, may lose consciousness with a red face.
Canth.
***

Anger (burning, deep).
Staph (long-standing), *Acon* (sudden unexpected rages), *Hep sul, Ign, Nux vom.*
Alternating despair and fits of rage at own performance, and others, and circumstances, may impede athletic performance. *Cer serp.*
Breakers of things who fly into rages at seemingly no provocation, seem like small children. *Cim.*
Unstable women with frequent rages and concomitant problems, unable to settle into life routine. *Ign.*
Intolerant coaches, trainers, senseis, may improve their performance immensely by taking this remedy. *Nux vom.*
Red face with bulging eyes and ugly personality, either a sportsperson or a coach, may be mellowed considerably. *Stram.*
Hypercritical, furious with loud shouting, may attack physically, a nightmare person to others in a group, a boss from hell, sees only his own viewpoint and unable to relate to others, closed-minded. *Ver alb.*
Deep brooding fury in a would-be achiever or frustrated person. Wastes time and energy on rage rather then intelligently working on improving his situation. *Staph.*

Focussed on revenge for real or imagined injustices, rage inhibits proper performance. May move into his own world in his own mind. May be alienated and may become violent. May turn against his own society. *Staph.*
***

Anger, exhaustion, remorse.
Lively person steadily gets worse with outbursts, low threshold, pounding heart, legs feel like logs of wood.
Phos.
***

Angry with himself.
Dissatisfied, hates people, repulsive, thinks he is dying, hears stepping in his head.
Aloe.
***

Anguish, terrible.
No end is in sight, complete despair, utter heartbreak.
Sweet chestnut. (Bach).
***

Anti-social.
Too shy and timid. *Mimulus (Bach).*
Very pretentious. *Vine (Bach).*
***

Anxiety (see also Apprehension, Stress, Fear, Phobia).
Arg nit, Ars alb, Gels, Lyco (in anticipation of something scary, demonstration, competition), *Sil.*
Fear of death, panic palpitations, cannot face the idea of performing or competing. *Acon.*
Forthcoming scary event. *Arg nit.*
Agitation, no confidence, depression, cyclical fears, believe they are ill and so unable to perform. *Ars alb.*

Intense fear of future level of performance. *Calc carb.*
Anxiety about being slow, ineffective and performing poorly, time seems to pass too rapidly as an event approaches. *Cocc.*
Trembling fear, so scared that physical performance is obstructed, nothing calms them as the moment approaches. *Gels.*
Thoughts become too fast and too intense, and terrify the patient to the point of being unable to participate in something. *Glon.*
Nervous about what is expected, sad, breathing trouble and may puff with fear, mood swings. *Ars alb.*
Stomach reaction to anxiety, diarrhoea before events, perhaps during them, and can severely curtail performance, especially in events such as martial arts gradings. *Kali carb.*
Philosophical fears of inadequacy, weather causes moods to fluctuate and change, depressions disrupt training schedules. *Phos.*
Brooding fears about performing, grudges, bad memories of past disasters, revenge clouds emotions. *Staph*.
Stammering anxiety, fear of darkness, afraid to perform. *Stram.*
Shaking clumsiness before a performance is required, un-coordinated. *Agar.*
A person with sudden mood changes, feels there is a lump in the throat, mental focus is not good, optimistic then disinterested. *Ign.*
Anxious about everyone else, deep fears for others' safety and wellbeing, burning heat and pains, bleeds easily,

poorly for storms, cannot function with adequate dedication and single-mindedness. *Phos.*
Free floating anxiety. *Aspen (Bach).*
***

Apathy.
Too little interest in the present, no spontaneity, no joy, resigned, flat in speech, monotonous, stagnant in endeavours, avoids engagement in activities, eats poorly, no vitality, tends to stomach ailments, lung problems and skin disorders. *Wild rose (Bach).*
Dreaming so much they never generate anything to cheer themselves up so they lose interest in living. *Ambra gris.*
In a reverie, hears things not there, may hallucinate, unable to make decisions, may not be able to respond normally to external stimuli. *Anac orient.*
Gone into another world inside their heads, lost contact with the world. *Hell nig.*
Sad and switched off, headaches, perhaps dizzy. *Mur ac.*
***

Apathy (living death) (see Nervous breakdown).
When a person descends into this state of apathy, much participation in life becomes impossible. Everything seems pointless, there is no more drive or energy. Life loses any attraction or significance whatever.
Chin, Nat mur, Phos, Puls, Sep, Mur ac.
Patient is unable to experience any pleasure at all, from the present situation. Dreams constantly of the past. *Ambra gris.*
Patient is in a reverie, can make no decisions, experiences auditory hallucinations, hearing voices in the head. *Anac or.*

Patient is in a stupor, displays no interest in anything at all, seems completely unaware of the surroundings, becomes worse when consoled. *Hell nig.*
Patient is deeply sad, irritable, apathetic, has headaches with dizziness, feels worse in damp environs. *Mur ac.*
Deadness. Patient seems to have died inside the head, mentally and emotionally, though bodily still functioning. *Ambra gris, Anac or, Hell nig, Mur ac.*
Patient experiences a deep melancholy, craves solitude, avoids company. *Sepia.*
***

Apologetic.
Steps back, self-demeaning, an apologist.
Pine (Bach).
***

Apprehension (see Anxiety).
Fear of possible or real events to come, imagination may work overtime visualising things which will never happen, mistakes, disasters, failures. *Lyco, Arg nit.*
***

Apprehension, melancholia, doubts, confusion.
Imagines all sorts of things happening, sad and weeping, focus on minutiae, overcautious, uses the wrong words and gets wrong message across, apathetic.
Calc carb.
***

Apprehensive from too much happening at once.
Many life-events are taking place, such as deaths, pregnancy, illness, re-locating, career changing, weddings, studying, tyranny of the system, court cases etc.
Arsen alb.

***

Approval needed all the time.
Has difficulty acting alone, needs the re-assurance of someone else, wants approval for actions.
Cerato (Bach).
***

Arguments in the head.
No peace of mind because of the clashing inside the head.
White chestnut (Bach).
***

Arrogance.
Arrogance can surface in those who deep down feel inferior, and not being able to accept this truth, they adopt an arrogant attitude in their efforts to impress others. It backfires, of course, and leaves the arrogant people unpopular, disliked, without support and not part of the camaraderie of the team.
Hypercritical, brooding, bitter people, become disliked and left out of the mainstream. *Lyco.*
Delusions of their own greatness is not shared by others, and they are not appreciated, and become fearful and insecure, making poor coaches and hopeless bosses at work. *Plat.*
Anxious, critical sportspeople, with violent tempers, rarely achieve much in sport and are shunned by their fellow sportspeople. *Ver alb.*
Authoritarianism is sometimes accompanied by an inability to control the first instinctive reaction, which may be violent anger, which is soon gone. Many people in Western societies have been raised with the idea that they need not take orders, but conversely they also want to exert

control over others. The result is that the undisciplined ones never benefit fully from coaching and instruction, while those trying to control and lead, experience huge frustration and anger. Both leadership qualities based on knowledge, and the discipline needed to rapidly follow instructions, are critical to good coaching and top performance. *Aur met.*

Certain people are totally antagonistic to any new ideas, becoming fearful, and displaying wild anger over trivialities. These people are stuck in their grooves, and soon get left behind in training methods and therefore in performance. They arrogantly declare that what they learned once is the only possible way to do things, although it clearly is not so. This situation is extremely pronounced in the martial arts, as well as in some entire Western cultures which suffer from kainolophobia. *Nux vom.*

***

Attention, ADHD, ADD.

Inability to concentrate, or attention deficiency, creates havoc in schools and households and on sportsfields. Diet and food allergies may be contributory factors. There may be a refusal to follow instructions from a person in authority, with rowdiness, disruption and fearlessness, coupled with emotional problems like jealousy. Since remedies need to be personalised, i.e. selected to match each patient, this book can only list a few remedies which have worked for other people, so that you can try them or research them in your own Materia Medica.

Lach, Tub bov, Tub av, Calc phos, Calc carb, Caps, Med, Anac, Aeth, Cann indic, Baryta c, Tarent hisp, Stram, Bell, Hyosc, Lyss, Cina, Plat, Zinc met, Sul, Lyco.
***

Attachment to things, excessive.
Inner centre not stable, impressionable, inner peace disturbed, seeks stability, superstitious, religious, clairvoyant, cannot break with past, forebodings, digestion disorders.
Walnut (Bach).
***

Aversions.
Athletes and business-people may frequently need to travel to other venues and countries, where they sometimes have little option about what is fed to them. Foods which they are unable to eat, may upset their performance. There are many remedies for aversions to various foods, far too many to list here, so only a very brief cross-section is mentioned. Consult a good Materia Medica for more.
To various foods. *Stan met, Colch.*
Beer. *Nux vom, Rhus tox.*
Bread. *China, Puls.*
Butter. *China, Carbo veg.*
Coffee. *Coff, Spig.*
Fatty foods. *Carbo veg, Puls.*
Kitchen smells. *Colch, Ipec.*
Meat. *Arsen alb, Bry, Sep.*
Milk. *Calc carb, Sep, Sil, Cina.*
Tobacco. *Ign.*
***

Awkward.

Clumsy in mind, as in body, stutters, ineffective,
inappropriate, not with it, lost, takes things the wrong way,
absent-minded, forgets, laughs and cries alternately and at
the wrong times, sad and argumentative, sits and stares.
Bovista.
***

B.
***

Backward, daft, silly.
Slow to understand, misses the gist, thoughtless and
childish, whines, mentally weak, forgets, imagines legs are
cut off, grief, feels the butt of humour, hides, holds hand
over face, idiocy.
Baryta c.
***

Begrudges.
Resents anything good among other people, begrudges
anyone good fortune, a spoilsport and grumbler, ungrateful
for anything, determined to wallow in self-pity.
Willow (Bach).
***

Belonging, no sense of.
Can feel no real reason to be there, feels out of place, does
not belong.
Cerato, Larch, Scleranthus (all Bach).
***

**Bereavement, emotional shock. (see Shock or Trauma)
(see Grief).**
A reaction of disbelief, showing signs of being completely
stunned, with yawning and sighing, may discount any
chance of good life performance. *Ign.*

Bereavement, grief (see Bereavement, Shock)
Nat mur, Puls, Ign, Aur, Kali phos.
A grieving person may feel things very strongly, be super-sensitive to slights, losses, deaths. They may remain silent about losses, isolating themselves, and can be the worse for any heat. This can preclude good life performance. ***Nat mur.***
Cardiac shock may be a result of bereavement, with heart attack, leaving the person faint and weak, bluish, with dilated eyes. ***Digit.***
A person may think of a death, go into shock, suffer fatigue, talk to himself all the time, mutter, show great fear with diarrhoea, have painful limbs, feel weak and too heavy. ***Gels.***
Blood pressure may drop, blood supply to organs will drop, resulting in tiredness, apathy, coldness, blue colour, nausea, thirst, faintness, shallow breathing, anxiety and possible confusion. So take grief seriously and understand that it may completely stop top performance for a while or even forever.
***

Bewildered.
Confused, not sure what is going on, wakes up a bit lost and uncertain, gloomy, cannot fix attention on things.
Aesc hippo.
***

Bi-polar disorder (extreme mood swings).
People are dependent upon a settled and focussed mind for good performance. When moods fluctuate, then so does performance.

Diagnosis may easily be incorrect, as mood swings can be prompted by various physical conditions, and occurrences in the life of the patient. The latter could include a host of relevant matters, viz. anything which can make one's emotions react, from foods to colleagues, work, wars, societal changes, spouses and more.

The physical conditions can include AIDS, brain tumours, head injuries, diabetes, epilepsy, lupus, Lyme's disease, multiple sclerosis, neurosyphilis, sodium imbalance, thyroid problems and more. These all need to be ruled out to make certain one is dealing with bi-polar disorder.

Treat symptomatically with homeopathic remedies which you can locate under the headings in this book.

Here are some very early warning signs, because the sooner treatment is begun, the less the severity of the depressions will be. The severity of a full blown, living death hell, where the sun can never reach, can not even begin to be understood by those who have never been there. The signs are:

Separation anxiety.

Tantrums.

Great irritability.

Oppositional behaviour.

Mood fluctuations.

Inability to concentrate for any time.

Times of incredible activity.

Impulsiveness.

Fidgety.

Being daft and clowning.

Thoughts wild and uncontrolled.

Aggression.

Grandiose ideas.
Eats masses of carbohydrates.
Takes stupid risks.
Depression.
Tired, no energy.
Self-esteem very low.
Cannot rise in the mornings.
Social anxiety and phobias.
Too sensitive, not normal.
***

These signs can be followed by a host of others, less
common, like speaking too fast, obsessions, compulsions,
forgetfulness, lying, suicidal ideas, paranoia, migraines,
self-mutilation, cruelty to animals.
***

As the disorder develops, specific characteristics emerge.
The main ones are:
Great fluctuations in physical activity and energy.
Considerable physical changes, weight, pains, etc.
Negative and powerful emotional plunging downwards.
Bad, unpredictable moods and pessimism.
Thought patterns change completely, disorganised.
Constant thoughts of death.
***

So stay alert, and react before the symptoms and warnings
become deeply embedded.
***

Biting people.
Rage with bizarre ideas, rituals, compulsions, may want to
stab herself, feels isolated, made worse by running water or
bright light, over-sensitive to sensory matters.

Hydro (Lyssin).
***

Bitterness, resentment.

For people unable to forgive, and certainly not able to forget, who dwell on their own past perceived bad luck. These are negative and unpleasant people.

Willow (Bach).
***

Blemish.

Obsession with a blemish becomes overwhelming, or too much.

Crab apple (Bach).
***

Bottled up feelings.

Cannot speak about problems, various fears, too much nervous tension, indifferent to people when ill, reacts sharply to atmosphere.

Phos.
***

Breakdown constantly feared.

Low self-image, feels stress will break him, too tensed up, fearful, anxious about things to come.

Lyco.
***

Brooding.

Despondent, sluggish, mentally slow, pessimistic.

Chel.
***

Bullying and insensitive.

For people who constantly try to enforce their wills on others, getting them to enter into things they do not want to

do. May stoke the ambitions of others unrealistically.
May be too hot all the time, especially at night, and also
have tantrums or yelling sessions. May be associated with
the suppression of skin symptoms. Skin may have
eruptions and itch and burn.
Sulph.
***

Broken up.
Feels as if in parts, scattered about, confused, has awful
nightmares.
Bapt.
***

Broodiness.
A pre-occupation with having babies, or making a home,
may impede life performance considerably.
Ign.
***

Bulimia (loss of appetite control) (see Hunger).
People need carefully balanced diets in order to function
optimally, and bulimia causes chaotic food intake, to the
detriment of general function.
Iod, Nat mur, Sul.
Permanent drive to stuff oneself with too much food, often
vomitting it all back out before it is digested. *Ant crud.*
Eating vast amounts whenever possible to comfort oneself
after emotional setback. *Ign.*
***

Burden, believes erroneously that he is a burden.
Cannot relax and blossom due to feeling a hindrance and
burden to other people.
Pine, Mustard (both Bach).

***

Burdened, unfairly.
Hard working, dedicated, serious, being suppressed and held down. Heart pounds with rage.
Aur met.
***

C.
***

Calamity expected, no reason.
Fearful for family and others, expects small ailments to grow enormous, thinks the worst may happen.
Red chestnut (Bach).
***

Camaraderie with others not possible.
Too aloof, cannot relax and chat easily.
Water violet (Bach).
***

Careworn.
Feel tired and weak, avoid all issues and confrontations, awake half-dead, aged too early.
Mag mur, Mag carb.
***

Changeability.
Emotions change all the time, adapting constantly but too much. May be weepy. Blocked nose, needs fresh air, needs coolness and rest.
Puls.
Changes of mood, rapid and unpredictable, fears, unable to act, tears, self-pity or blame, no resistance to the knocks of life, no anger, difficulty working.
Ign.

***

Changes personality or character.
Unreliable in character, may be someone else tomorrow.
Cerato, Scleranthus (both Bach).
***

Character traits (see also individual headings).
Certain traits can severely disrupt or completely destroy
lives and careers. A few of them are listed below, with
suggestions for their treatment. Traits can be there from
early on, or develop at any time in a person's life.
Sometimes they remain hidden for different periods of
time, or vary in intensity.
Overemotional. *Ign, Gels.*
Hyperactive and over-optimistic. *Sulph.*
Ultra-meticulous. *Arsen alb.*
Shy, retiring. *Puls, Nat mur, Sil.*
Wildly jealous. *Lach.*
Introverted, too much. *Staph.*
Impatient, irritable, always rushed. *Arg nit.*
Capricious. *Ign, Puls.*
Sullen. *Nat mur.*
Grumpy. *Nux vom.*
Ratty, loses temper. *Cham, Nux vom, Aur met.*
Authoritarian. *Aur met, Lyco.*
***

Chatting not possible.
Unable to relax and enjoy any banter or conversation.
Mentally and physically rigid. In a rush, everything too
slow.
Water violet, Impatiens (Bach).
***

Cheerful front.
For people who hide their real feelings behind a smiling face.
Agrimony (Bach).
***

Cherished surroundings lost.
Grief for being torn away from places, or people or work. Feels like heavy weight on the chest.
Caps ann.
***

Childish behaviour.
Sings, dances, shouts, over-sad at stories, confuses past and present, silly, childish gestures and arm-waving. Memory may fail, may not recognise people. Delirium, feels in a strange place.
Cicut vir.
***

Claustrophobia (with life).
A person who feels hemmed in, squashed, too crowded by factors and events in the life he is leading, can take remedies to alleviate the situation and help him back into the mainstream. He can also find counselling to assist him in outlook and perceptions, or he can change things in life to get rid of some of the offending problems, or he can do some of each.
Arg nit.
***

Cleans obsessively.
House-proud, feels dirty, disgust inside, ashamed of personal appearance, fusses.
Crab apple (Bach).

***

Clingy, weepy.
Must be consoled and pampered.
Puls.
***

Close, too close when speaking.
Does not want to be alone. Talks about self, saps your
energy, may be weepy.
Heather (Bach).
***

Closed-minded, dogmatic.
Tries to control others, categorises everyone, does not
allow others to be individuals or human, joyless, angry,
obsessive, tense with mental strain. Arrogant.
Rock water, Beech (both Bach).
***

Commanding others.
Must command, must lead, over-ambitious, over-
enthusiastic, impatient.
Vine plus Vervain plus Impatiens (all Bach).
***

Complacent, no urgency, just sits.
Wild rose, Clematis (both Bach).
***

Complaints quashed.
His own mind prevents him from voicing what is amiss.
Centaury, Agrimony, Oak (all Bach).
***

Complains constantly when ill.
Willow, Gorse (both Bach).
***

Comprehension so slow, can't understand.
Must be alone, sits motionless, weeps, cannot laugh nor
maintain proper conversation.
Ambra gris.
***

Compulsive.
Uncontrollable habits.
Crab apple (Bach).
***

Concentration (see Attention).
Focussed activities with no concentration must fail. Focus
and concentration need to be restored to establish a good
level of focussed activity.
People, active, struggling to concentrate, to maintain
attention. *Aeth, Sil.*
Intellectually exhausted, with memory loss, showing
indecision and low focus. *Anac.*
***

Concerned about others, too much.
Constant worry and circular thoughts about the safety of
people one knows.
Red chestnut (Bach).
***

Condescending.
Overpowering, controlling, self-righteous.
Vine, Rock water, Water violet (all Bach).
***

Confidence (gone).
Confidence in oneself is of enormous value to people. It
starts in the planning, progresses to the preparation and is

essential in the execution of the chosen activity, and without it, a person flounders.
Lyco.
***

Confrontation avoided at all costs.
Dutiful but deeply vexed, great annoyance.
Mag mur.
***

Confusion.
Fight or flight goings on, depressed, hypochondria, feels guilty, deep concern with salvation and church, anger, staggering.
Lil tig.
***

Confusion about the future is intolerable.
Must think he has control and security, worry, agitation, especially at night.
Arsen alb.
***

Confusion, shrieks.
Convulsions possible, cramps, twisted face, shrunken appearance in bluish face, cramps.
Cup met.
***

Confusion, unreal feeling.
Slow-motion of everything, feels as if he experiences all stimuli from someone else's body, as if he were in that body using its ears, nose, eyes and senses.
Alumina.
***

Conscientious, over-conscientious, obstinate.

Feels pushed around, doubts, can be spiteful, can be courageous.
Sil.
***

Consolation, aggravates grief and disappointment.
There may be headaches, stammering, eye problems, skin and digestion disorders, hots and chills.
Nat mur.
***

Consolation constantly sought.
Sufferer is never consoled, never feels better, seeks more consolation, revels in it.
Willow, Chicory (both Bach).
***

Consolation makes everything worse.
Disdainful, condescending attitude.
Water violet (Bach).
***

Conspiracy, imagines.
Fears there are conspiracies all around. Anger and hatred felt for the supposed perpetrators, cannot rejoice in the joys of others, suffers in the mind, intolerant.
Holly (Bach).
Lives in fear of possible conspiracy against him, fears insanity.
Cherry plum (Bach).
***

Constricted feeling (squashed).
A person needs to breathe easily and move easily, relaxed and free of fetters. An emotional sensation of being squashed, limits ability.

Cact.
***

Contempt.
Contemptuous of everything and everyone, disobedient, fixed ideas of unhappiness, feels persecuted, dislikes work, amazing fantasies and daydreams, writing and speech disjointed or faulty, tries to hurt feelings.
China off.
Contempt with anxiety and moroseness.
Ipec.
For self, for actions now despised, feels a failure and unclean.
Crab apple (Bach).
***

Contradiction (flies into rage if ideas contradicted).
People fail to learn new techniques, and may fail to work well in a team. People unable to accept instruction and contradiction probably need treatment. Bigotry and rage impede activities.
New ideas make them murderously angry. *Nux vom.*
Cannot hold back rage at change or development, people can be taught this on a wide scale, hence ideologies, becoming outdated, bigotry, being left behind, the so-called "dinosaur", kainolophobia. *Staph.*
Intolerance to contradiction.
These people cannot live and let live, are often from unforgiving backgrounds and were severely restricted as children. *Aur met.*
Such people are closed minded, or narrow minded, seeing only one possible course of action. They may be

intelligent but totally critical of anything that does not conform with their ideas. *Lyco.*

These people may be good workers, are tense, and cannot accept any changes. They are short-tempered and will always argue, so have trouble progressing. They are a nuisance to have in any group you are teaching or coaching. *Nux vom.*

***

Contradictory symptoms.

These may be quite odd, and there are numerous examples. One example may be feeling very hot but insisting on being covered with a blanket. Logic is defied. Appears after great disappointment or grief.

Ign.

***

Contradicts non-stop.

Quarrels all the time, never satisfied.

Ruta.

***

Control, emotional control absent.

Feels different, unruly and unwanted emotions and thoughts inside, impulses, mania, delusions, visions, subconscious mind awakening with nightmares and rages.

Cherry plum (Bach).

***

Coping, cannot cope anymore.

Normally confident people, now overwhelmed with too many things and too much responsibility. Despondent, cannot get into action, cannot be effective.

Elm (Bach).

***

Conversation blockage, unable to chat.
No self-assurance, awkward, fears failure, no ambition, fear of poverty and disasters, fear of rejection.
Mimulus, Larch (Bach).
***

Cravings (this is only a short list, there are many more remedies to help you stop overeating).
People need careful planning and control over their diets. Cravings may disrupt proper diet. The remedies listed below may offer some assistance with eating properly.
Acid foods. *Sep, Nat mur.*
Alcohol. *Sulph, Lach.*
Beer. *Kali bich, Aloe.*
Bread. *Ferr phos.*
Butter. *Merc viv, Ferr phos.*
Cakes. *Carbo veg.*
Coffee. *Nux vom, Carbo veg, Cham.*
Eggs. *Sulph.*
Fatty foods. *Nit ac, Nux vom, Sulph.*
Fish. *Nat mur.*
Fizzy drinks. *China, Lyco.*
Fruit. *Sul ac, Mag carb.*
Hot drinks. *Arsen alb, Lyco, Sab, Eupat, Med.*
Hot food. *Lyco, Chel.*
Ice cream. *Calc carb, Ver alb.*
Indigestible foods. *Calc carb, Alum.*
Meat. *Allium sat, Calc phos.*
Milk. *Abro, Phos ac, Staph, Mag carb.*
Oysters. *Lach, Calc carb.*
Salty food. *Nat mur, Carbo veg, Arg nit.*
Smoked meat. *Calc phos, Caust.*

Spicy food. ***Sep, Nux vom, Hep sulph.***
Sugar. ***China, Lyco, Nat carb, Arg nit.***
Wine. ***Zinc.***
***

Crawling round floor after leaping out of bed like a madman.
Haemorrhages, grief, worries, forgetful, unable to recognise people.
Acet ac.
***

Creatures creeping in the dark, ghosts.
Nostrils flare, drinks cold water and vomits, upset stomach, chest constricted.
Phos.
***

Crisis, still in shock.
Rescue Remedy (Bach).
***

Critical of everything.
Overenthused, overcaring, too fervent, overconscientious.
Beech, Chicory, Vervain (Bach).
***

Cruel.
Tyrannical, aggressive, demands obedience, dictatorial, without compassion.
Vine (Bach).
***

Crying does not happen.
Feels she must cry, but nothing ever happens. So sad.
Amm mur.
***

D.
***
Day dreaming instead of working.
Unmotivated, wishing for happiness, imagines joy in the
future, disconnected from present, low adrenaline and
thyroid, poor circulation. Absent-minded.
Clematis (Bach).
***
Dazed, not with it.
Unfulfilled, wandering thoughts, trance-like, spaced-out,
sad, former happiness gone. Delayed shock.
Clematis, Star of Bethlehem (both Bach).
***
Dead inside, perhaps from grief.
Emotionally numb, completely apathetic.
Phos ac.
***
Decisions, too scared to make them.
Some people are so uncertain of themselves, and untrusting
of their own judgement, that they need others to help and
reassure them all the time.
Cerato (Bach).
***
Defects, certain she has critical defects.
Feels unable to proceed and cope because of real or
imagined defects.
Crab apple, Cherry plum (mental) (both Bach).
***
Defiant when given instructions.
Answers back angrily, responds with defiance or
antagonism to normal instructions or orders.

Vine, Vervain, Chicory (all Bach).
***

Delay impossible, gets frantic.
Lonely, isolated, superior attitude, drives others rather than lingering with them, cannot be hindered, rude, manic, abusive.
Impatiens, Vervain (both Bach).
***

Delegate, completely unable to.
Has to do the job herself, has to make sure it is done as she wants it to be. A perfectionist. Other people too slow.
Vervain, Impatiens (both Bach).
***

Delirium, mania, fears of rats.
Can't keep still goes from place to place, fidgets incessantly, tries to injure herself, feelings of impending evil, visions of rats and mice terrify her, weak willed, suspicious.
Cimi race.
***

Delusions (see Winning).
Feels everyone has lost confidence in him, that he will fail in everything, that he does everything wrong.
Aur met.
***

Demands on him excessive.
Made worse by disappointment and bottled up failure, possible burning of intestines from mouth to anus, headaches, blurred eyes, nausea, various disorders.
Iris vers.
***

Dementia.

The onset of dementia will interrupt activities at an ever-increasing rate, until they cease altogether, forever, quite possibly.

It is customary to attribute dementia to Altzheimer's disease, but there are many other disorders which also cause dementia, some of them haltable or curable. Homeopathic remedies should be applied symptomatically. Here follows a brief description of the disorder and some causes.

Dementia is a neurological disorder, affecting the ability to think, speak, reason, remember and move. Sometimes aspects get worse with time and are incurable, but sometimes they are reversible, or can be effectively treated at some point. The most common causes are Altzheimer's disease, Vascular dementia, and Lewy body dementia. A person may have one, two or three of these at the same time. Several more common causes are also listed below.

Altzheimer's, involves loss of nerve cells in parts of the brain, associated with clumps of protein in brain cells. First sign is forgetfulness, followed by language deterioration, reasoning, understanding, and finally the ability to care for themselves. Risk increases with age.

Vascular dementia frequently follows a stroke, when arteries to the brain are obstructed, with sudden onset usually, although sometimes onset can be slow, affecting thinking, language, walking, bladder control, and finally vision.

Lewy body dementia occurs when abnormal round bodies, called Lewy bodies, develop in the cells of the brain, and it may be that all the above forms of dementia are related.

Frontotemporal dementia affects the lobes responsible for social behaviour, resulting in rudeness and inappropriate behaviour.

Huntington's disease is hereditary, starting with mild personality changes, developing into jerks, clumsiness and weakness, followed by dementia.

Parkinson's disease sufferers may become stiff and shaky, with tremors, speech impediments, shuffling gait, developing into dementia.

Creutzfeldt-Jakob disease is rare, linked with eating beef from cattle with mad cow disease (bovine spongiform encephalopathy).

Inability of the liver to eliminate certain medications, may lead to dementia, which may be reversible.

Metabolic deficiencies, in the form of hypothyroidism, hypoglycaemia, or pernicious anaemia, can all lead to personality changes and dementia.

Chronic alcoholism can lead to dementia.

Severe emotional problems or setbacks can lead to dementia.

Infections such as meningitis, or encephalitis, syphilis or AIDS, can lead to dementia.

Once diagnosis is complete, then various forms of dementia can be controlled or reversed, but it is critical to know and understand the cause before it can be treated.

Unfortunately, memory loss and confusion, apathy, forgetfulness and depression, are so often lumped under one heading, usually Altzheimer's, that treatment is not effective.

***

Depression (see Melancholia).

Depression may seriously disrupt or destroy schedules.
Arn, Ars alb, Calc carb, Kali phos, Nux vom, Sep, Onos.
This really needs an experienced homeopath to select a
constitutional remedy, but in the meantime you may have
success with these remedies.

Person has experienced too many setbacks. *Staph, Ign.*
Disgust with life, with sport, with everything. *Aur met.*
Mentally overstressed and overworked. *Kali phos.*
Solitary brooder, unable to discuss or share problems. *Nat
mur.*
Post-natal depression. *Sep.*
Inhibited, sensitive type, feels unable to cope and falls into
depression. *Ambra gris, Ign.*
So tired, indifferent, cannot care anymore, life seems
pointless. *Phos ac.*
Lost confidence, fears doing things, timid now. *Lyco.*
***

Depression with fear.
Anxious and depressed, fears of never being cured of
anxiety. *Arsen alb, Lyco.*
***

Despair.
This condition may remove all motivation and desire to
take part in life, or alternatively may remove any
motivation for success.
Acon, Ars alb, Bry, Calc carb, Nux vom, Sep.
***

Despondent, whining, peevish.
Frightened, cannot be alone, suffers a lot, dizzy on arising.
Ant tart.
***

Destructive rage.
Cannot use setbacks constructively, feels inferior, full of envy.
Staph.
***

Detail, obsessed with.
Feels dirty in mind, secretive, feels flawed, fears all contaminations, obsessed with trifles.
Crab apple (Bach).
***

Determination to succeed.
Success constantly jeopardised by oversensitivity to outside influences and pressure from others. Adverse circumstances and ridicule undermine drive forward.
Walnut (Bach).
***

Devastated.
From shock, bad news, sorrow, upset, funeral, failure, inability to face up to the problem or occurrence, accident, injury, fear, panic, loss of calm. Cannot focus attention.
Rescue Remedy (Bach).
***

Devotion to duty not appreciated.
Feels lost and misunderstood, full of resentment, singing ears.
Kali carb.
***

Devotion to loved ones drained out.
Indifference to others, withdrawal, self-pity, yellowish skin with bloated abdomen a characteristic.
Sepia.

***

Diplomacy absent.
No understanding that others have different opinions. A possible perfectionist when others are not. Impatient and rushed when others may be relaxed. Thinks he is perfect while others are full of shortcomings.
Beech, Impatiens, Vine, Holly, Vervain (all Bach).
***

Direction in the passage of life.
Fails to get going, has ideas, dreams, education, intellect, but is unable to put it all into action. This remedy, together with daily affirmations and work, will encourage actions and activity which can be dramatically life-changing.
Germanium.
***

Direction, keeps losing it, coming back again.
Needs help to maintain path in life.
Walnut (Bach).
***

Direction, sense of direction fails, lost.
Not sure where he is, confused.
Glon.
***

Disappointment (huge).
Ignatia.
Bitter, indignant with how his affairs have gone, considers the world unfair and against him, "knows" everything else will be the same. *Staph.*
Frustrated and disappointed with life and affairs, suffers the same thoughts endlessly repeating themselves, going

round and round. Cannot be optimistic about life or anything else. ***Thuja.***

Disappointed in love, thinks it is only him, feels he is at fault, feels unworthy and badly treated. Loses confidence in his abilities to overcome difficulties, so unable to be good at life tasks. ***Nat mur.***

Surly instead of friendly and outgoing, angry with people and the world, disappointed with life, certain his life will fail too. ***Sil.***

***

Disaster, constantly feels disaster is on the way.
Calc carb.

Lives in fear of possible natural and financial disaster.
Calc fluor.

***

Disconsolate, cries for nothing.

Hopeless, despondent, fatigued, confusion of letters and syllables, Spoonerises.
Caust.

***

Discontent, failing ambitions.

Has a calling or mission, cannot decide on the correct path or assess own abilities. Wants to achieve but not take responsibility, unfulfilled, joyless, frustrated, not able to insert meaning into his activities.
Wild oat (Bach).

***

Discontent, permanent feeling of.

For no reason, just has a feeling that all is not as he wants it, grumpy with the situation, may complain, wants to talk.
Bism.

***

Discouraged (see Nervous breakdown).
After experiencing difficulties with little or no progress,
stress, bad times with poor performance. *Ambra gris.*
Mentally exhausted from struggling, worn out, no drive to
live. *Kali phos.*
Gentian, Elm (both Bach).
***

Disdainful.
Unable to cope easily with vexations, defensive over-
reaction to things, vengeful, jealous, hateful, rages,
competitive, plots, easily insulted. Wants beauty and
perfection in everything. Intolerant, racist, typically
expects performance from others while stopping progress
with criticism and evaluation. Feels persecuted. Difficult
to focus on life tasks with all this going on in the mind.
Holly, Beech, Vine (all Bach).
***

Disgruntled person.
Full of resentment, anger, bitterness, and irritability.
Cannot wish others well, jealous, unkind, a spoiler of good
spirits, never satisfied or contented.
Willow (Bach).
***

Disharmony, cannot tolerate.
Unable to have any aggression around him.
Agrimony (Bach).
***

Disillusioned, frustrated.
Angry, abusive, disappointed, self-control weakened,
palpitations.

Ign.
***

Dislike, of self.
Overflows with self-reproach, sees own sins and failings, stifled by introflection, desires punishment sometimes, perfection-orientated, remorse, temper, not properly focussed on life.
Crab apple, Pine (both Bach).
***

Disobedience to authority.
Loves rhythmic music, intense, rushed, resistant to work, impatient and grumpy.
Tarent hisp.
***

Dispirited, mental fatigue.
Tired and low, no desire to work, may forget to do things, forgets schedule, has trouble keeping to schedule, unenthusiastic, does not feel as if success will be achieved, sad.
Arn, Gels, Ign, Lach.
***

Displeasure and capriciousness at everything.
Impatient and angry.
Ipecac.
***

Disregarded, so angry.
Not being cosseted, not getting desired sympathy, becomes angry and shows it.
Puls.
***

Distracted, unsettled, influenced.

During a time of change and adjustment. Needs to settle and be calm and focussed.
Walnut (Bach).
***

Distraught about welfare of others.
Excessive worry about others can lead to excessive worry about their own well-being, nervous fears, sleeplessness, vertigo, nausea, trembling possible.
Cocc indic.
***

Disturbed mind.
Denies any disorders but full of vexations and resentments, no inner peace so cannot tolerate outer disorder, cannot be happy in the present anywhere, anxious about future, tends to drugs, seems cheerful. Difficulty in seriously focussing on occupation.
White chestnut, Agrimony (both Bach).
***

Dogmatic.
Rigid in outlook, fixed in ideas and opinions, closed-minded to new information, resistant to change.
Rock Water (Bach).
***

Dominance and power.
Must accomplish things fast, pent-up energy, violent and excitable.
Tarent hisp.
***

Dominating position.
People who dominate others, abusing their positions to enforce their own ways and ideas, taking no consideration

of the views of others, giving instructions all the time. They are like small children trying to enforce their own ways over everything.
Vine (Bach).
***

Doubts everything and everyone.
No self-assurance, defines self by opinions of others, uncertain, doubts own memory and estimations, anxious, feels body is weird, hesitant speaking, no clarity.
Gentian, Cerato (both Bach).
***

Dread, fear, anxiety.
Haughty, circular thoughts all night, half dead in the mornings, aversion to new things or changes, talks in sleep, hypochondria.
Lyco.
***

Dread, nervous dread about tomorrow.
Exhausted and overwrought, prolonged strain.
Kali phos.
***

Dread, of what may happen.
Deep seated fears, superstitions, religion, apprehension, acute terrors, intense phobias, fragility, unstable, no nerve power, threatened, violent. Life difficult.
Aspen, Rock rose (both Bach).
***

Dreams.
Bad dreams can debilitate people, causing disruption in life.

Terrifying dreams. ***Acon, Alum, Ars alb, Calc carb, Nat mur, Phos, Puls, Thuja.***
Dreams of murder. ***Arn, Nat mur.***
Dreams of dead people. ***Ars alb, Thuja.***
Dreams of being chased. ***Sil, Sulph.***
Dreams he runs so fast but cannot escape, or go anywhere, just seems stuck. ***Cad met.***
***

Dreams transformed into reality.
This remedy seems to tip the scales, enabling people with ideas and dreams to actually put them into action, and to follow them through. A must for people stuck in a rut.
Germanium.
***

Driven to high standards of work.
Personal integrity very high, tense, worried, drives non-stop, muscles seize up in neck etc.
Nux vom.
***

Drive for accomplishment.
This is so strong that all personal needs and requirements are put aside, resulting in various disorders and aches and pains all over.
Rock water (Bach).
***

Drive gone.
No exuberance, apathy, resignation, serves at own expense, feels guilty, low Vital Force.
Centaury, Wild rose (both Bach).
***

Duality, two people inside her.

Very fixed preconceptions, someone behind all the time, or inside, sees other faces in mirror, hears voices from the dead, fears and religious mania, screams, may swear and curse, full of contradictions, unintelligible speech, laughs at the wrong times, cruel, anti-social, suspicious, fear of paralysis or poisoning.
Anac.
***

Dull, slow, weak, sad.
Anxious about the future, despondent, dulled senses.
Digit.
***

Duty owed to him.
Requires everyone to conform to his ideas and values. Selfish, offended, disapproving.
Chicory (Bach).
***

Dying, convinced he is.
Refuses to do anything, dying, forgets things, thick head.
Agnus cas.
***

Dying, illogically expecting to die shortly.
Loses interest in all worldly matters, not dying at all, it is only in the mind.
Phyto.
***

E.
***

Eating compulsion.
Will not stop eating. Logic has no power over the compulsion.

Crab apple (Bach).
***

Ecstasy, gaiety.
So many ideas, over-excited, acts on ideas, changes swiftly from joy to gloom and back, irritable, rolls around in anguish.
Coffea crud.
***

Emotions, cast aside for pragmatism.
Little affection given, little rage shown, people refined, helpful, major internal conflicts may lead to disorders, especially of the internal organs.
Chel maj.
***

Emotions.
Chinese medicine and the emotions.
As in homeopathy, Chinese medicine sees the system as being a unity, with all aspects interlinked and communicating with each. However, Chinese medicine has been around for thousands of years longer than has homeopathy, or the recent arrival of Western medicine. More for interest than for use, although it may cast some light upon basic conceptions of health, I am very briefly touching on how Chinese medicine might approach the matter of emotional obstructions to life performance. It is worth bearing in mind that Chinese medicine is generally very effective, and has also kept so many people alive that the population of China is the biggest on earth.
***

Fears of real and imagined things, weak willpower causing poor performance, insecurities about own abilities and

acceptance by others, aloof from other people. The kidney function is treated.
***

Too tired to train, no enthusiasm for life, mental restlessness and poor concentration, depression, insomnia leaving him exhausted, despair of ever achieving anything. The heart function, and its health, is addressed.
***

Anger, resentment, frustration, irritability, bitterness and inappropriate rages causing poor performance. The liver function is in disorder.
***

Worry, dwelling on problems, mental overwork, thoughts going round and round, inability to plan and properly execute life tasks. Spleen is suffering and needs attention.
***

Grief, sadness, indifference to the self, to life, to other people, general malaise and lack of interest. Lungs are treated.
***

In each case one can see how much the interactive effect of the physical and mental is taken into account. In Western allopathic medicine, and psychology, there is a tendency to imagine that symptoms are isolated occurrences and can be treated alone.
***

Emptiness of the heart, after loss.
No emotions left.
Star of Bethlehem (Bach).
***

Enlarged objects of vision.

Things seem far bigger than they really are, his sense of spatial and size judgement is defective. Line of thought lost at the slightest interruption.

Berb vulg.
***

Enmity, chronically repressed.
Escalating tension, annoyance, fear of losing control, serenity impossible.

Impatiens, Cherry plum, White chestnut, all together (all Bach).
***

Enraged with the injustice of the system.
Fears losing reason and control and acting in violent ways, mania, destructive rage, escalating intolerance, paranoia.

Holly, Cherry plum, Vervain (all Bach).
***

Enthusiasm gone.
Full of apathy, no drive, no interest, perhaps after a big shock.

Opium.
***

Enthusiasm, too much.
Over-excited, hates being alone, may brood.

Ver alb.
***

Envy/hatred.
Vexed, suspicious, malicious, indignant.

Holly (Bach).
***

Escapism, mental, unable to focus on life.

Longing and wishing, pleasant delusions, spaced-out smiles.
Clematis (Bach).
***

Exam, grading, trials terrors.
Rescue Remedy (Bach).
***

Example setting.
Always trying to be the example that belittles all others, rigid, unmoving, closed-minded, a martyr, ruled by theories.
Rock water (Bach).
***

Excessive behaviour patterns.
Shrieks, convulsive laughing with violent weeping, talks too much but shuns people, spasms and convulsions, nausea, foaming at the mouth, uses wrong words, may bite and attack, tears things, mimics.
Cup met.
***

Excitement (too much leaves her ill).
Some athletes, either before, or after an event, or when involved with other groups or different clubs, coaches and courses, can become completely ill and demoralised by pure excitement. The illness may be physical, or emotional, or mental, or a combination of these in different intensities.
Bell, Acon, Arg nit, Aur, Graph, Nat mur.
***

Exhilaration, persecution, bliss, untidy.

Moral senses blunted, craves obscurity, senses death, feels covered in bugs and worms, jealous, thinks others are talking about him.
Cocaina.
***

Exploited people.
Kind, hard-working people, who cannot stand up for themselves.
Centaury (Bach).
***

Exultation, exaggeration of imagination.
Intoxicated, hallucinating, mania and grandeur, inappropriate laughter and giggling.
Can indic.
***

Eye-contact, avoids.
Has specific fears, concrete things now and in the future, fears rejection, imagines specific problems.
Mimulus, Aspen (both Bach).
***

F.
***

Façade.
Always has a brave face or appearance to hide inner turmoil. Acts carefree to conceal inner suffering of the mind.
Agrimony (Bach).
***

Failure anticipated in everything planned.
No confidence in possible success, expects and therefore finds failure in many activities.

Larch, Mimulus (both Bach).
***

Failure, fear of.
Some people have such a fear of failure that they never try anything at all. They may lack any confidence in their own abilities.
Larch (Bach).
***

Fanatical.
Extremes, too much effort, too much energy put into something, goes past normality, cannot give it a break. Hyperactive on something. Typical of religious fanatics.
Vervain.
***

Fate, terrified of possible fate.
May shoot self, hates life, hates food, hates bathing, forgets to perform toilet unless reminded, angry at any attention, lovesick, may talk in rhymes. Crude, greedy, vulgar.
Ant crud.
***

Fatigue, incoherence.
Incomplete sentences, stuttering, confusion, wavering.
Can sat.
***

Fault-finding obsession.
Cranky, irritable, reacts against any demands on him, thumping heart, anguish, hot.
Nit ac.
***

Fearful of imagined or possible diseases.

People with a tendency to be flabby and overweight, and who get colds easily. Forgetful.
Calc carb.
***

Fears (acute, sudden, disrupting).
If fears are long-standing fears, ongoing over a long period of time, perhaps decades, disrupting life completely, then have a look at the section on Phobias.
Sudden fear of death. ***Acon, Arsen alb.***
Terror of darkness. ***Acon, Lyco, Stram, Phos.***
Panic in crowds. ***Arg nit, Lyco, Acon.***
Sudden fear of the dead. ***Acon, Ars alb, Lyco.***
Sudden pre-occupation with fatal disease. ***Phos, Sep.***
Fear of other people. ***Acon, Ars alb, Aur, Lyco, Nat mur, Rhus tox.***
Terrorised by storms. ***Rhod, Nat mur, Phos.***
Fear of making speeches. ***Lyco, Arg nit.***
Stage-fright, anxiety in front of people. ***Arg nit, Gels, Ign, Lyco.***
Paralysing fear, free-floating, unattached to a specific cause. ***Opium.***
Afraid of animals. ***Hyosc, Stram.***
Imagines burglars threatening all the time. ***Arsen alb, Nat mur.***
Claustrophobia with geographical area, or certain people, or house, office, country, occupation, family. ***Arg nit.***
***

Fervent, too much.
Tries to influence everyone else to own ideas, self-righteous, fanatical, too much of a hurry, ecstatic, hysterical neurosis.

Vervain (Bach).
***

Fighting, violence, disrupts everyone.
There is plenty of information available about these primitive types. Parts of the brain, the civilised, well-mannered parts, properly socialised, sometimes do not function, or have not developed at all. Sometimes they have been damaged by disease, miasms, smoking, alcohol, drugs, blocked arteries or accidents. The people cannot behave themselves, and have limited self-discipline. They are dangerous on roads, and bad to have in the employment situation. They say the wrong things at the wrong times, to the wrong people, and antagonise others. The problem relates to an evolutionary situation, in some instances, with throwbacks to earlier, undeveloped brains, suddenly appearing. In other cases the person may be the latest in a long line of undeveloped creatures, still close to "ape-men" or Neanderthals, but with speaking ability.

Humans have not been out of primitive savagery for very long, and display it all the time around the world. Road rages, aggressive driving, air rages, robberies, murders, assaults and war-mongering, are among visible manifestations of primitivism. Laws, without enforcement, can in no way control the violent impulses in savages, and a complete societal move, especially involving the complete media, schooling, prisons, and everything else in society, needs to be activated, to prompt evolution in a positive direction. Of course, civilised violence is often necessary to halt uncivilised violence.

Various tranquilizers and behaviour altering medications are available, which sometimes keep the inner cave-man at bay. Homeopathy offers some assistance in controlling such people, and helping them to work off frustrations in sport.

People with violent and aggressive dispositions, who frequently suffer depression at night. *Hep sulph.*

Jealous, suspicious, full of antagonism as adults, fighting everyone as children. *Hyosc.*

People who blame others for everything, agitated, . shouting, screaming, anxious, irrational. *Ver alb.*
***

Fixated.
Rigid minds in rigid bodies, overwrought, hypertension, hyperthyroidism, sees disagreement as a challenge to exert own willpower over others. Best to avoid these types. *Vervain (Bach).*
***

Fixed behaviour patterns.
Some people do not learn from mistakes. They are closed-minded, and repeat behaviours which are harmful to themselves. It seems to defy all logic, when these people constantly repeat behaviour which blatantly harms their own affairs. They may sometimes be termed "left-brainers". They do not see the whole picture, only the small matter within their focus. *Chestnut bud (Bach).*
***

Fixed in routines and surroundings.
Will not change, indolent, not well, lax.
Caps.
***

Floating on air.

Feeling of floating, can't think, light, feels stupid, cannot keep thoughts.
Asarum europ.
***

Flying (fear of).
Impulsive, rushing people, on the way to an event suddenly are incapacitated by fear of flying. *Arg nit, Acon.*
***

Follower.
Not energised from within, derives energy and motivation from others, must follow.
Cerato (Bach).
***

Foreboding.
Plagued by the idea that something bad is going to happen. No rational basis for this, but terrible fears, especially at night.
Aspen (Bach).
***

Fortitude absent.
Discouraged, never blames self for weakness, sees insurmountable obstacles, little faith.
Gentian (Bach).
***

Fragility, emotional.
Fears looking foolish, fears of losing mind, pre-occupation with ailments, fiddles and wastes time, self-pity, weeping, poor memory, religious mania, night fears.
Calc carb.
***

Frantic activity and rage.

Tension and energy far too high, over-reacting, mania, internal pressures lead to outbursts, sudden fears, possible stammering.
Stram.
***

Fulfilment out of reach.
Skills, talent and drive are present, but the path ahead is never clear, clouded with indecision and uncertainty.
Cannot select the way forward.
Wild oat (Bach).
***

Futility.
Overwhelmed by the futility of it all, unrecognised, undermined, low self-image, disturbed, may become cruel.
Anac orient.
***

G.
***

Gargoyles laughing and shrieking at him.
Talks flat out, spits, bites and tears at the hideous faces pestering him, wants to hide, weeps, quarrels, moans, ferocious.
Bell.
***

Getting going, unable to get movement, stuck.
Sometimes people know they need to do things, to get into action, and they know what to do, but are unable to raise the strength to actually do things. They put off starting until the next day, constantly.
Hornbeam (Bach).
***

Gloom.
Deep dark gloom descends like a cloud with no reason.
Mustard (Bach).
***
Grief (see Bereavement, Shock).
Nat mur, Puls, Ign, Aur, Kali phos.
For people who feel things very strongly, are super-sensitive to slights, losses and deaths, but remain silent about their grief, isolate themselves, and feel worse for any heat. Often resistant to comfort and may feel guilty about relief from suffering. Chronic, long-term. *Nat mur.*
Acute, sudden grief. *Ign.*
Effects of bad news. *Star of Bethlehem (Bach).*
General physical and mental illness after grief, with anger, blame, longing, pains, cravings or averseness to salt and sea air. Blocked nose. *Nat mur.*
Spiteful great rages, postnasal drip, worse in stormy weather, resists consolation, blame, childhood humiliations return to haunt her, all triggered by grief. *Nat mur.*
***
Grievance, but unable to voice it.
Racing mind, propelled forward, ecstatic, tries harder and harder to enforce own ideas. Thin and intense.
Vervain (Bach).
***
Grim, determined to survive.
After emotional setbacks, no humour, no relaxation and pleasure.
Nat mur.
***
Grudges held.

Goes round and round in anger, sleepless, critical, unmoved by apologies.
Nit ac.
***

Guilt, so great it obstructs life.
Aur met, Ign, Nat mur, Puls.
Excessive feelings of guilt, fate, rage, jealousy. *Lach.*
For those who despair because they feel so guilty, but remain fastidious about everything. *Lil tig.*
For those who feel very guilty, resigned, sad, loving, helpful, and need sympathy to be effective. *Puls.*
Free-floating guilt complex. *Pine (Bach).*
***

H.
***

Half dead, apathetic.
Mentally exhausted, no energy or drive at all.
Olive (Bach).
***

Hallucinations (see a doctor).
When your mind causes you to see things which are not there, you know you have a problem. Hallucinations may totally disrupt your life.
Excited, visual or auditory hallucinations, possibly feverish, with prostration. *Antipyrine* if available.
Visual and auditory hallucinations, grandeur, hilarity and anxiety, conversations, shouting. *Cann indic.*
Visual hallucinations, sees all sorts of things which are not there. *Hyos nig.*
Agitated, afraid of the dark, terrified of visual hallucinations. *Stram.*

Spectres and visions, monsters, terrible gargoyle faces, all glare and pull faces at the patient, who fights and rages and bites at them. ***Bell.***
***

Harmony craved.
Weak, broken down feeling, no peace of mind.
Mag carb.
***

Harsh.
Aggressive, critical people, with chest, bronchial, sinus, sciatica, asthma, arthritis disorders, hyperthyroidism.
Kali iod.
***

Hate, simmering.
Injustice seethes, smouldering resentment, blaming, shirking, vindictive, no forgiveness, fallen from grace, enjoys misfortunes of others, feigns illness.
Holly, Willow (both Bach).
***

Hates other humans.
Works self up into states of violent anger, morose.
Ledum.
***

Head feels huge.
Irritable, oversensitive, head feels as if in water and greatly enlarged, must loosen clothes, clumsy.
Bov.
***

Hesitancy, uncertainty.

Indecisive, changes choices all the time, thoughts all over, no clarity. Can be hormonal. Gait may be uncertain. Non-stop, "Shall I, shan't I"?.
Cerato, Scleranthus (both Bach).
***

Highly-strung.
Exaggerated drive, palpitations, irritation, rush.
Nux vom.
Loquacious, too excitable.
Cimi race.
***

Home, must go home.
Cannot stand people around him any more.
Bry.
***

Homesickness.
Making functioning effectively almost impossible.
Ign, Nat mur.
Nostalgia, regrets, fear of the future, longing for the past. Loses contact with the present, Vital Force weakens.
Honeysuckle (Bach).
***

Hopelessness.
No faith, feels nothing can be done, no hope at all.
Gorse (Bach).
***

Hormone related hysteria.
Rage, noise, emotions.
Asaf.
***

Hostility, smoulders.

Kept suppressed for years, overt compliance.
Willow (Bach).
***

Humiliation.
It is not easy for people who are angry, resentful, feeling
their boundaries have been violated, to function optimally.
This may especially be the case after an episiotomy.
Staph.
***

Humility and empathy absent.
A taskmaster who criticises others, sees only his own
viewpoint, demands discipline from everyone, isolated.
Beech (Bach).
***

Hurry.
Hurry can stop a person from thinking, considering and
weighing up, so paradoxically, hurry can cause years of
wasted time and effort. A wise man once said, "Don't just
do something. Sit there".
Cannot stop rushing, will not stop and consider. ***Arg nit.***
Overworked, not organised, overactive, nervous. ***Nux
vom.***
Rushes. ***Acon.***
***

Hyper-active.
Rushed, compulsive, excitable and impatient, violent,
aggressive, suppressed anger, suicidal, disorders of the skin
and breathing apparatus.
Arsen iod.
***

Hypersensitivity (to almost everything, touch, pain, noise, light, exercise etc).
Violent, intense (usually), splinter-like pains, pus in sores or wounds. Better for heat and lying down. *Hep sulph.*
Becomes angry over noise, smell, talking, light, is always grumpy. *Nux vom.*
***

Hypochondria (convinced they are ill).
Imagined illness completely obstructs life activities.
Wants to die, thinks he is so sick. *Aur met.*
Broods and does not discuss (mostly stomach) problems.
Nat mur.
Terrified of any little symptom, convinced it is fatal. *Phos.*
Indifference, denies he is ill, must be alone, nightmares, afraid of illness and sudden death.
Arn.
***

Hysteria.
All the energy wasted in hysteria, and looking silly at the same time, combine to detract from an optimally functioning situation.
Aur, Gels, Ign, Lach, Nat mur, Puls, Sep.
Hysterical grief may be uncontrollable and need time to settle (see Bereavement). *Ign.*
Over-dramatisation, being a "drama queen", may be a symptom that all is not in order elsewhere in the person's life and mind, self-image etc. It has no place in an effective person's life. *Mosch.*
Rescue Remedy (Bach).
***

Hysterical excitement.

There can be all sorts of physical manifestations and reactions. Patient may feel a cloud is enveloping him.
Cim race.
***

I.
***

Identity lacking.
Does only what conventions dictate, or what others expect.
Centaury (Bach).
***

Idiocy.
Weeps, spasms, pains, sees imaginary creatures, may leap out of windows, fearful. Likes animals.
Aeth cynap.
***

Idiocy and moral depravity.
Titters, wrings hands, feeble minded, gabbles mindlessly and rages at people, masturbates without shame, bites at people, deceitful and wants to be alone, hates music.
Bufo.
***

Ill-treatment from others leads to grief.
Bad manners, misbehaviour, causes sadness or grief.
Colch aut.
***

Imagination, stagnant.
Anticipation dead, no more promise, religion has died in the person, Vital Force is weak and immune system weak. No endeavour to improve matters.
Wild rose, Gorse (both Bach).
***

Imposing love and rules on other people.
Some people think they can rule anyone they decide to
love, and they try to impose strict conditions and rules.
They forget that others do not want to be ruled and
controlled. They are frequently deeply hurt when not
accepted.
Chicory (Bach).
***

Impossible to please.
Spiteful, rude, bad-tempered even with self.
Cham.
***

Impulses, violent, stammering.
A smelly person all round, with weakness and trembling.
Merc.
***

Impulsive, aggressive, shuns people, checks things.
Disorder caused by forced inactivity, or shock or
disappointment, compulsive checking of things repeatedly,
very hot body with palpitations.
Iod.
***

Incoherent.
Switches subjects all the time. Indifferent, staggers, drops
things, shudders, restless, sings, hilarious, morose,
stubborn, throws things, cannot learn new things nor can
he work.
Agar.
Incoherent, obscene, over-excited and obsessional, hard
done by, may be senile, has conversations with the dead.
In his own world.

Hyosc.
***

Inconsolable.
"Locked in" grief, sighing, overwhelms entire existence, feels completely abandoned.
Star of Bethlehem (Bach).
***

Indecision.
Cannot chose any direction, seeks a mission to fulfil, life seems meaningless.
Scleranthus, Wild oat (both Bach).
***

Indecisive when alone.
Needs confirmation from others, wants advice, always wants guidance.
Cerato (Bach).
***

Indifference to everything.
Patient no longer cares whether life is important or not, or even what happens to him, or anyone else.
Chin, Nat mur, Phos, Puls, Sep.
***

Indifference to loved ones.
Feels weary, has no interest in family or loved ones, shooting pains in head, dark rings under eyes, nausea, pot-belly perhaps, dry cough, itchy. Better when active or in action. Cannot conceal thoughts, snappy, cries. Bottled up despair. Torpor, wants to hide.
Sepia.
***

Indignation.

Questions enrage him, may be very embarrassed.
Coloc.
***

Indolent.
Dull, slow, indifferent, uninterested, fears of darkness and ghosts, sluggish, stupid, lazy.
Carbo veg.
***

Inert from exhaustion.
System tired out, too exhausted to move or think.
Olive, Hornbeam (both Bach).
***

Inertia.
All aspirations submerged, dormant, no interest.
Hornbeam, Wild rose (both Bach).
***

Influenced too easily.
Outside influences remove the ability to make own decisions, immature, unable to feel certain of own decisions, needs assurance from outside.
Walnut, Cerato, Wild oat (all Bach).
***

Initiative too low, sits and worries.
Fails to get things done, concentration low.
Graphites.
***

Injustice.
The patient is seething with deep rage, may feel deeply wronged, perhaps bypassed. The sense of unfairness can leave a person sick with anger, wasting energy on futile rage, unable to settle to proper functioning. The immune

system may weaken, the appetite may diminish, and general decline in performance may come about. It is not wise to put off treating rage, as ill-health may result, as well as stomach ulcers. *Staph.*
Vervain (Bach).
Incensed.
Caust.
***

Insanity, brutal, kleptomania, avoids people, violent convulsions.
May fall over backwards. Shuns any human contact. May have awful seizures with foaming at the mouth.
Absinth.
***

Insanity, fear that it is happening, in someone's head.
Thoughts seem without logic, and the mind seems to be falling to pieces. *Cherry plum (Bach).*
***

Insanity looming large.
Haunted, sick of life, overtly fine, feels insanity coming on to him.
Merc sol.
***

Instability, extremes of emotion.
Deep inside there is a lack of a stable core for endeavour or relating to other people.
Erratic emotions alternating with erratic physical expression. *Scleranthus (Bach).*
Seeks affection but does not return it, sullen tendency.
Chicory (Bach).

Seeks attention but fails to verbalise inner needs, talks a lot about personal problems. *Heather (Bach).*
Emotions unstable and swinging. *Elm (Bach).*
Inner needs make her feel shame and embarrassment. *Crab apple (Bach).*
Glides over the real problem, cannot confront it. *Cherry plum (Bach).*
Core too sensitive to every little influence, reacts too much and too readily, needs strengthening and stabilising, needs some shielding. *Walnut (Bach).*
***

Insults, dwells on ancient ones.
Feelings easily hurt.
Staph.
***

Intellect overrules emotion and being human.
Makes his own rules and structures, shuns people, lives in a world of the mind.
Kali bich.
***

Interest in learning new things gone.
Withdrawal, no more development, stagnated, heavy, immovable.
Wild oat, Mustard, Hornbeam, Chestnut bud, all together (all Bach).
***

Interpersonal power craved.
Critical, discontented, very irritating people.
Nit ac.
***

Intimidated.

Cannot say no nor stand up for own rights.
Centaury (Bach).
***

Irrational.
Too much on the go, irrational, unreasoning rage at
inability to cope makes things worse. Nervous tics,
spasms, jerks, involuntary gestures, grinding teeth.
Emotion overrules rational thought, juvenile behaviour
results.
Cherry plum (Bach).
***

Irresolute.
Can not act without approval from others, passive, no
drive.
Baryta carb.
***

Irritability if things seem slow.
Certain people think that everyone else must do everything
at their pace. They seem unable to understand that people
do not do all things in a rush nor at the same speed. People
do different things at different speeds, depending on
familiarity with the matter, and many other factors.
Rushing, irritable people can be very irritating to other
people.
Impatiens (Bach).
***

**Irritability with nausea, bearing down pains inside
body.**
Sepia.
***

Injures own skin.

Rage and aggression towards others is turned on the self.
Holly, Willow, Cherry Plum, all together (all Bach).
***

Injustice, incensed.
Tense people who are extremely stressed because of the
injustice they see around them. They try to persuade
others to see things as they do. A sense of injustice can
pervade their entire lives.
Vervain (Bach).
***

Insecure, emotionally.
Feelings of others do not count, self always first, must
voice injustices, misfortunes and betrayals. Fixed on
certain topics of conversation.
Cerato, Mimulus, Heather, Chicory (all Bach).
***

Intolerant and critical of how others do things.
People who just cannot grasp that others do things
differently to what they do. They are irritable and cranky
and do not understand others at all.
Beech (Bach).
***

J.
***

Jabbers mindlessly.
Impatiens, Agrimony, Mimulus (all Bach).
***

Jealousy.
An emotionally unbalanced patient may experience terrible
jealousy, unfounded suspicions, unclear thinking, and even
fear poisoning.   The   pressure   and   desperation   for

achievement in some areas of society, can lead to non-achievers becoming quite unhinged. Examiners or team selectors may become the objects of hate, and coaches may be blamed for poor performance by athletes, when in fact they themselves are not up to par. Suspicious people may suspect intrigue among others is keeping them down, or that racial bias is holding them back
Lach, Apis mel, Hyosc.
***

Jubilant, too much, overdone.
Nerves and mind affected, laughing mania, whistles, shouts, jumps and dances, tries to kiss everyone, laughs then weeps, suddenly sings.
Crocus sat.
***

Jumpy.
Gets frights all the time, nervous, starts.
Calend.
***

L.
***

Laughter, maniacal.
Incoherent person, hallucinates, jumps, terrible dreams.
Bell.
***

Laughter uncontrollable, followed by rage.
Scolds and laughs hysterically.
Mosch.
***

Laziness.

Imagines good future, rather than working for it, goes into reverie, floats. Unable to apply himself hard and regularly. No diligence in pursuit of goals and hopes
Wild rose, Clematis, Hornbeam (all Bach).
***

Learning from mistakes, impossible.
Repeats same errors. Seems compelled to continue in same pointless cycle. Cannot recognise the error of his ways. Unable to see himself in perspective, as others do.
Chestnut bud (Bach).
***

Let down.
Joyous anticipation is followed by terrible let down and disappointment. The grief can affect the moods which swing, and there can be physical reactions like rigidity, cramps and partial paralysis, twitches, pains and sleeplessness.
Ign.
***

Lethargy.
Weary, no interest, trifles hinder him, unable to learn, judgement poor, no staying power. No great achiever.
Hornbeam, Wild rose (both Bach).
***

Liar.
Lies all the time, even when it is obvious that others know. Will not stop lying. A compulsive disorder.
Heather, Chicory (both Bach).
***

Lies for attention.

Opinionated, expects appreciation, self-pitying, offended, feigns illness for attention, hypochondria, false accent to conceal real self, manipulative, histrionic, false.
Heather, Chicory, Willow (all Bach).
***

Limbs, feels he has too many.
Septic, poisoned blood, fevers, stench, vomitting, terrible stench from toilet, ulcers, painful bones, chills.
Pyro.
***

Limbs feel severed and scattered about.
Feels broken up, rolls about trying to collect separated limbs, they talk to each other, may feel double, cannot exert himself, hopeless.
Bapt tinc (Canadian thistle).
***

Loathes self.
Disgust for self, feels unclean and purges self of uncleanness, hidden vices and addictions, rituals and behaviour patterns fixed, erroneously views body as distorted or ugly.
Crab apple (Bach).
***

Longing, nostalgia.
Constricted chest, longing for loved-ones or places, suffocation from sadness.
Aur met.
***

Loquacity, too much.
Silly, yaps too much to cover inner nervousness.
Ambra gris.

***

Losses suffered.
Terrible grief, overwhelms personality, great depths of
sadness and depression.
Star of Bethlehem (Bach).
***

Love, unable to give, blockage.
Cannot show feeling of love.
Chicory, Holly (both Bach).
***

Lunatic behaviour in bursts, dangerous, mad.
Cannot be looked at or touched, especially children. Life
is unbearable, falls in love easily, loves moonlight.
Ant crud.
***

M.
***

Malcontent.
A malcontent can never settle and enjoy life, nor allow
others to do so. Consequently such people never excel in
activities they constantly put down, and among people they
constantly criticize.
Never satisfied, vengeful, throws juvenile tantrums,
disruptive. ***Cham.***
Broods over past slights and sorrows, instead of thinking
and planning ahead. Focus is on bad elements of the past
instead of happy elements of the future. ***Staph.***
Stubborn and stupid, changes ideas all the time, contradicts
what has just been decided or said, not reliable, demands
things then rejects them. ***Cina.***
***

Malicious.
A liar, fabricates malicious stories, aggressive, full of hate, suspicion and jealousy.
Holly (Bach).
***

Mania (insanity, nervous breakdown).
The patient may suddenly be overtaken by religion, and indulge in frenetic religious activity, exhibiting obsessive compulsive behaviour with great exultation. Life performance drops off. ***Stram, Melil.***
Signs of mania which are visible to others and indicate that proper concern is called for, although treatment may be almost impossible to the over-excited person:
Great energy, restless, tireless, obsessed with the new idea.
Rapid speech, often incoherent.
Clang associations, fixating on words with similar sounds, repeating them at every opportunity ad nauseam.
Judgment of life is poor, socially and financially, grandiose and inappropriate.
Clear change in sexual behaviour is possible, with hitherto hidden orientations appearing from nowhere.
Thought patterns alter, becoming disjointed and difficult to follow, disorientated and dislocated, racing furiously.
Mood swings begin, from hostility to loving, ecstasy to depression, inexplicably.
Perceptions alter, delusions appear with paranoia, religious fervour and missionary zeal take over.
It is important not to confuse mania with short-term projects. Mania overtakes the entire sufferer's existence in a permanent fashion, bringing about a complete alteration of the mind, changes of friends, divorce. Short projects

need fast thinking, energy and different perceptions, to drive them to fruition, after which the person reverts to "normal".
***

Manipulative, sly.
No care for others, self-opinionated, does good works for recognition and gratitude only, ulterior motives, feigns illness, invents pains, attention-seeking.
Chicory (Bach).
***

Martyr.
Spiritually active, seeks self-mastery, tries to inspire others, self-denial, rituals, punishes self, seeks purity of the soul, immense inner strain, suppressed normal human characteristics.
Rock water, Chicory (both Bach).
***

Matter-of-fact people.
All strong emotions quashed. Disorders surface in many forms because of this.
Kali carb.
***

Melancholia (see Depression, Winning, for information on the destructive wrath of melancholy).
Melancholia kills normal abilities.

Such people are sometimes visionaries, who have to be perfect in all their many undertakings, yet who feel they are never appreciated. Those around them rely on their strength, yet they feel unrecognised, and they strive for appreciation, and never feel they achieve it, so become critical and angry, and display sycotic (miasm, see section

on miasms) traits, and then depression sets in. *Aur sul.*
Also of use, Nat sul, Thuja and Med.

As they harbour unrealistic expectations, melancholic people suffer constant disappointment, and become insecure because of repeated disappointments, persuading themselves that all matters will disappoint, so becoming secretive. Disappointment has dogged them since puberty, suicidal feelings often lurk in their minds. Because of chronic disappointment with love affairs, women sometimes develop cancers or uterine problems and men grow cancers of the prostate gland. *Aur mur nat.* Other useful remedies are *Arg mur, Zinc mur nat, Cup mur nat, Baryta mur nat, Plat mur nat, Plumb mur nat.*

***

Below are a few characteristics of melancholy people, together with some possible remedies.

Broods, cries, oversensitive. *Ign.*

Fearful, avoids people, in a daze. *Gels.*

Lacks confidence, fearful, timid, emotional, discouraged, self-pity evident, indecisive, weak, better after eating. *Kali phos.*

No happiness, the same negativity day after day, the same brooding unhappy thoughts, unspeakably saddened by life and events. *Lach.*

Self-confidence gone, feelings of worthlessness, morose, authoritarian, loses thoughts. *Lyco.*

Fantastic visions of achievements, compensating for imagined childhood abandonment, not achieved. *Aur iod mag.*

Utter desperation for admiration. *Aur iod sul.*

***

Visions of life are not achieved because of the failure of others, real or imagined, but he does not complain, and goes from doctor to doctor becoming progressively more ill, is diagnosed as depressive suicidal and hypochondriacal. Anger and restlessness are clearly present in the mind. *Aur mur.*

Abandoned by life partner, melancholic, depressed, suicidal. *Aur iod nat.*

Terror of abandonment by friends and family, even the imagining of it causes illness and disorders, melancholia. *Aur iod kalin.*

Melancholics fear being abandoned if they are not the best, or not something, and think they will lose the safety and protection of the herd if they do not achieve. They need a herd, and when not achieving what they think they have to, they become deeply distressed and ill. *Aur iod calc.*

There is a desperate need and desire for admiration, appreciation, from close family and loved ones, and when it is imagined that it is not there, deep distress results. *Aur sul kalin.*

The melancholic person craves protection, is desperate for safety and frantic for security, must be appreciated. *Aur sul calc.*

The patient feels like an orphan, which he may or may not be, and can only overcome the feeling by achieving appreciation and admiration. He feels a failure at achieving this. *Aur sul mag.*

The patient has a very intense feeling that his own abandonment is at hand, so forms over-strong attachments to those seen as supporters. He tends to be emotional, loving, very bored and must travel. The most important thing in his life is a partner, but he is always plagued by insecurity, feeling the partner is about to leave. *Aur iod.*

A person with all the traits of those needing Aur iod, yet seeing the family, or group, as the most important thing in life, yet feeling insecure and fearful all the time in case the family leaves, afraid the family may steal from him, may benefit from *Kali iod.*

There is a desperate desire for appreciation, and perhaps adulation, in relationships, with fanatical efforts to get recognition, and fears of being abandoned. *Aur sul nat.*

Patient suffers a deep, debilitating fear that friends and family will withdraw love, and bewails his possible fate, thinking friends will rob him. *Aur mur kalin.*

No-one and nothing lives up to expectations, causing constant disappointment, with intense and deep need for a feeling of protection. *Aur mur calc.*

Unable to trust, full of suspicion, the patient looks for back-stabbers and robbers. He may be a leader who mistrusts all the supporters so wants to control everyone, needing strict order and meticulous arrangements, always wondering if enough has been done, and also experiencing some guilt that it might not have been. But conversely, there is a dislike of fastidiousness, with obsessive-compulsive disorders and mood disorders, sycotic and syphilitic characteristics. *Aur arsen.*

Extroverted, lovely people who are hard workers and very creative, but so longing for love that they search incessantly. They may be tubercular, and never find the love they seek. *Aur phos.*

On a permanent search for love, but only in relationships, these types suffocate people, never finding love for more than a fleeting moment. *Aur phos nat.*

Extremely creative people, very overly demonstrative in efforts to be loved, strong and very lonely, very giving. *Aur phos mag.*

Constantly expecting abuse for being the best, and for accomplishing things. Expects antagonism for being a visionary, and this paranoia is very evident, followed by possible delirium and psychoses. *Aur brom.*

Terrible insecurity, especially in private matters, needing to be creative and trying to hide problems in hard work, fearing abuse. *Aur brom nat.*

Very worried, even as adults, that their parents, or protectors, will abuse them, because they are not the best, and they try to overcome these feelings with hard work. *Aur brom calc.*

Mixed up with frustrated creativity, fears of abuse and a persistent feeling of orphanhood real or imagined. *Aur brom mag.*

Over-sensitive people always getting hurt, trying not to hurt others, avoiding close relationships, introverted because of this, and when hurt they fall into a depression and become hypochondriacal. *Aur chrom.*

A greedy person, wants immediate gratification, aggressive to those who do not provide it, will break the relationship, anger is channelled off via arm and leg movements. *Aur fluor.*

Strong feelings that protectors are not doing what they should to satisfy needs, also need an outlet for creativity, aggression towards parents, employers, friends,

disappointment, depression, but fear of losing safety and protection. *Aur fluor calc.*
Patient experiences anxiety, feels inadequate, desires to be the best, and has visions of achievement undermined by visions of inadequacy and failure, and feels unable to manage, but aims high. *Aur carb.*
Inadequate in relationships. *Aur carb nat.*
Disappointed, unfulfilled, hypochondriacal, blames others and circumstances, imagines undefined danger all around, fears imaginary threats. *Aur nitricum.*
Note: There is considerable speculation and thought about whether different cultures experience the same problems. It seems unlikely that people brought up in certain Western cultures, expecting all their deepest desires and needs to be supplied by others, including parents and governments, will be the same as people who are brought up to be thankful for what they have. The author is a Soke, teaching various aspects of Eastern cultures and philosophy, and teaching the principles of being able to function completely without support, or conversely, being able to contribute fully to the greater good without expecting personal rewards in return. The typically Western idea of thinking that one is special, and entitled to having everything given to one on a plate, may possibly be construed as a distortion and morbid phenomenon, resulting in some symptoms of melancholia and other emotional and mental disorders.
***

Melancholic.

Joylessly introverted, dark cloud covers mind, no aim,
stifled, feels hopeless, withdrawal from life, no energy, no
stamina, poor sleep.
Mustard, Gorse, Sweet chestnut (both Bach).
***

Memories, too sad.
Faith gone. The state which made happiness, and
experiences to grow and develop, seems gone forever.
Lack of resolution, stuck in mourning.
Honeysuckle (Bach).
***

Memory (filing and storing information).
Life may become almost impossible or difficult for people
who forget things all the time.
Forgets names, specific information. **Anac or.**
Mind wanders, cannot keep on track. **Baryta c.**
Loses train of thought, temporary amnesia. **Cal seg.**
Forgets parts of, or mixes up sentences, may have
nightmares. **Kali brom.**
Cannot keep mind on an idea, like a butterfly. **Kali phos.**
Forgets names of people and places. **Lues.**
Memory is like a sieve, needs notes. **Med.**
Lapses, struggles at jobs, forgets. **Nux vom.**
Generally forgetful in work, the home, shopping etc. **Phos
ac.**
Daydreams, forgets what he is doing. **Sil.**
Names and events escape him altogether. **Sulph.**
***

Mental arguments.

Unable to release thoughts. Cyclical, no finality, apprehensive, interacts with others constantly in the mind, caught by the cycle.
White chestnut (Bach).
***

Mental confusion (nervous breakdown).
Life activity becomes impossible under these conditions. The patient has no hope, and feels like two people, with part of the body detached, indifferent to all things, with no concentration span at all. *Bapt.*
Patients experience delirium to stupor, jealousy and suspicion, blame others for everything, talk only about work, are exhibitionists. *Hyos.*
Slow, dimwitted people, un-reactive to events, indolent, appear not to hear or see, worse for heat and better for fresh air. *Opium.*
Psychological upheaval appears to be happening. *Gels.*
***

Mental control, losing it.
Irrational with dangerous impulses, faster and faster out of control, fears and phobias, anxiety. Possibly murderous and violent.
Arg nit, Cherry plum (Bach).
***

Mental conversations, sometimes replay continually.
Self-image sometimes vulnerable.
Lyco.
***

Mental fatigue.

This can result in unfounded terrors, memory loss and
disappearance of any confidence, which leads to the
collapse of normal life skills.
Tragedy and fright cause awful dreams, shouting in the
sleep, depression. *Lach.*
Yawning, sighing, crying, ball of tension inside patient.
Ign.
Trembling and fearful of all things. *Gels.*
Inert, prostrate, cannot move or act. *Arnica.*
***

Mental troubles following sickness or injury.
Suspicion, green vomit, painful bloat, gurgling bowels,
asthma, cough. *Nat sulph.*
***

Mind power gone.
Switches subjects, forgets, deceiptful, quiet, restless travels
around, acts on whims, does weird things.
Arg met.
***

Mind vacant.
Exhausted so quickly, heedless, weak intellect, makes
mistakes, forgets.
Ammon carb.
***

Misfortunes of others affect her too much.
Morose, impatient, indignant.
Coloc.
***

Mistakes, will not learn from.
Inattentive to lessons, impulsive and stupid, foolishly does
things which caused trouble in the past, repeats mistakes

constantly, lack of reasoning power, poor socially, cannot change adverse routines. Unable to alter ineffective routines.
Chestnut bud (Bach).
***

Mixed up emotions.
Illogical fears and dreads, faltering, gives up, expects failure in all things, low self-esteem, memory fails, weeps, irrational conclusions to matters, incoherent, stays in bed.
Arg nit.
***

Mixed feelings.
Rebellious, passionate, suppressed rages from abuse, guilt deep down, explodes at criticism, loves beat and rhythm.
Carcin.
***

Monsters in the mind, patient bites and hits at them.
Bell.
***

Mood swings.
Imbalance, constant changing, alternates, hormonal disturbance, insecure feeling, may stagger, stomach ulcers, tyrants sometimes.
Scleranthus, Mustard (both Bach).
***

Mood switches, restlessness.
Joy switches to spite, laughter turns to rage, happiness turns to destruction, cannot wait for anything.
Tarent Hisp.
***

Moon problems (full moon problems are quite common but rarely spoken about).
The moon may affect various things within the human system, causing disorders and disruption.
Any person exposed to the moon may experience emotional and physical problems. *Ant crud, Arg nit, Thuja.*
Waxing moon disorders. *Thuja, Staph, Alum, Arsen alb, Clem erec.*
Waning moon problems. *Thuja, Dulc, Iod.*
New moon. *Kali brom, Staph, Caust.*
Full moon. *Sulph, Phos, Nat mur, Calc carb, Cina, Sep, Sil.*
***

Mother hen constantly worrying about others.
Always anxious about the safety and welfare of other people.
Red Chestnut (Bach).
***

Muddle-headed.
Slow to comprehend, can't think of what to say, anxiety.
Merc.
***

Murderous desires.
Very violent impulses and intentions.
Cherry plum (Bach).
***

N.
***

Nags.
Critical, unsympathetic, irritated by people.

Beech (Bach).
***
Names, calls things by wrong names.
Diosc.
***
Negatives, sees only.
Thinks it's all caused by others, fails to see one's own
contribution to a negative situation, resentful, dissatisfied,
digestion seriously affected, ulcers and vomit, irritable
colon, hypertension.
Willow (Bach).
***
Nervousness.
A burning off of nervous energy may sap the abilities of
any person. A certain amount of nervousness is good for
functioning, but more than that depletes energy supplies.
Arg nit, Ign, Lyco.
The person is weak in resolve, needs support and
encouragement to perform to full ability. This remedy is
particularly good for blonde, plump women, emotional and
weepy, but works for most other people too. ***Puls.***
***
Nervous breakdown (see Discouragement, Apathy).
Effective function becomes impossible under the
circumstances.
Patient suffers utter trembling nervous exhaustion, feels
frozen, becomes incoherent. ***Agar.***
Something has set them back emotionally, they keep
crying, become weak and avoid people. ***Ambra gris.***
Patient is suicidal, perpetually sad, exhausted, fearful, has a
poor memory, becomes very irritable. ***Anac or.***

Patient is suicidal, crying and sad all the time. ***Ant crud.***
Patient experiences permanent disgust with life, fears own suicide, has huge rages. ***Aur met.***
Patient is aged, stiff, quiet, thin, depressed, sad, worse at night but better when warm. ***Caust.***
Mental capacity declines noticeably with the patient becoming angry about it, he hates noise and his memory becomes poor. ***Cocc.***
Patient becomes completely withdrawn, seems incapable of effort, memory seems gone. ***Fluor ac.***
Patient alternates physical tiredness with considerable excitement, followed by further tiredness, after long worry and fearfulness, loss of love. ***Hyos nig.***
After trauma the patient withdraws and becomes silent. ***Ign.***
Patient has financial worries and nightmares. ***Kali brom.***
Mental overstrain causes discouragement, indecisiveness and collapse of willpower, coupled with no physical energy at all. ***Kali phos.***
Deep melancholy pervades the patient. ***Lil tig.***
Self confidence is completely gone, so the patient cannot consider activity at all, and wants to be left in peace. ***Lyco.***
Indifferent, self-centred and brooding patient, becomes very sad. ***Nat mur.***
Completely burned out and overworked, the patient cannot make an effort anymore, and becomes disgusted with life. ***Nux vom.***
Patient can no longer think, goes into a mental torpor, cannot face mental challenge and finds memory adversely affected. ***Phos ac.***

Complete indifference, wants solitude, cannot take coldness, no energy at all, grumpy. *Sep.*
***

Nightmares.
Nightmares can be exhausting and disturbing for some people, detracting from their overall abilities and achievements.
Stram, Kali brom, Hyosc.
Horrors, terrors and panics. *Rock rose (Bach).*
***

Noise (hypersensitive to).
Certain noisy environments will make it impossible for hypersensitive people to perform properly. Remedies can make it more tolerable for them.
Bell, Chin, Acon, Nux vom, Sep, Therid, Strych, Kali phos.
Noise penetrates every fibre of the body. Therid.
***

Noise, unable to tolerate.
Spiritual, dignified, proud, religious arrogance, no easy friendship, cannot tolerate any humiliation, does not need others, hates noise, may get rigid with muscular stiffness and be poor in activities because of it.
Water violet (Bach).
***

Nosey.
Wants to get into every detail of other people's lives, tries to bind others to themselves, opinionated, controlling, digs in other people's goods, horrendous to have around one.
Chicory, Heather, Vervain, Cerato (all Bach).
***

O.
***

Obligations to loved-ones dropped.
Feels indifferent to the needs of closest family and friends,
feels no love for them.
Sepia.
***

Obstinate, heedless of others.
Capricious, unsatisfied.
Kreos.
***

O.C.D. (Obsessive compulsive disorder).
This is a long, slow disorder to cure, possibly taking years.
It is completely unlike some other mental disorders which
can often be switched in a day. Long term benefits may be
achieved by using the following remedies.
*Lach, Ac nit, Anac, Nat mur, Arsen alb, Thuja, Sab, Stan
met, Med.*
***

Offended (takes offence too easily).
The person who wastes time, focus and energy on taking
offence, will be at a disadvantage to the person who lives
above the pettiness of others. Remedies can sometimes
bring peace of mind to people, so allowing them to devote
their full energies to their lives.
Alum, Aur, Sep, Nux vom, Lyc, Ars alb.
Offended by petty things, feels humiliated and wounded,
very irritable, craves stimulants and fats. *Nux vom.*
***

Omens.

Seem to substantiate numerous fears and possibilities of things going wrong, irrational, deeply insecure, manic, obsessive, thinks he offends everyone.

Arsen alb.

***

Omnipotent, feels.

Demanding, threatening, manipulative, haughty, arrogant, zero empathy, no respect, disruptive, socially disastrous, consequently a poor team person.

Vine (Bach).

***

Opinions not allowed to be expressed.

Social or work circumstances force him never to express his opinions, so inner conflicts arise, with anger, coughing, tightening of the chest.

Agrimony (Bach).

***

Opportunity missed.

Too timid, indecisive, fearful, unconfident, no faith, negative.

Gentian, Cerato (Bach).

***

Order and efficiency.

Must have control at home and at work, wants to belong, domineers, geared to achievement.

Chel.

***

Outbursts of rage.

Holly (Bach).

***

Outraged.

Much too fervent about views, totally self-righteous, can never be wrong, overwrought, frantic, may be thin and intense.
Vervain (Bach).
***

Over-burdened.
Too many things have to be done.
Elm (Bach).
***

Over-compliant.
Fearful of annoying someone, suppresses feeling, frightened.
Acon.
***

Over-identification with the sufferings of others.
Feel they are the other person, suffer as much or more, no separation between their own sufferings and those of others, almost a telepathic identification. Frightened people with fantasies, monsters, spirits, sometimes thinking they have a terrible disease growing inside them. Phantom noises in the closet. May need re-assurance and hugs. Incredible flights of imagination. Rubbing or massage often helps a lot. When their imagination is channelled, these people can become very productive.
Phos.
***

Over-stressed, key-up.
Irritable, uptight, aggressive, intolerant of others, perhaps from drug abuse, forgetful of events, rages and door-slamming, crying.
Nux vom.

***

Over-sympathetic and over-critical.
Sees the worst scenario, cries, timid, full of suspicion.
Caust.
***

Overwhelmed by life.
Joy gone, brooding, sad, dispirited, negative, disturbed,
unable to focus.
Lach.
Overwhelmed and scared stiff. Feels a complete failure.
Kali carb.
***

Overwrought, desperate to comply with requirements.
Panicky, doing his best, struggling.
Asarum europ(ae)um.
***

Own problems discussed in great depth.
These people can go into great detail about their own
health and problems, to the boredom and frustration of
everyone else. They talk endlessly about themselves at
every opportunity.
Heather (Bach).
***

P.
***

Pain, fear of.
Allium cepa.
***

Panic.

Athlete suddenly experiences the fear of death, perhaps about performance or competition, or even selection for a team or event.
Acon.
The mind may go completely blank when the person needs to perform mentally or physically, or even with words.
Anac or.
***

Paranoia.
Feels someone is always there, sufferer is influencing, sensitive, conscientious, dreams of the dead, generally worse at full moon and better after exercise.
Thuja.
***

Paranoid fears.
Imagines threat, over-reacts to it, failing impulse control, highly competitive, rage, indignation with others, delusional.
Holly, Cherry plum (both Bach).
***

Past, lives in the past.
Some people dwell on memories and lose contact with the present, to a greater or lesser extent. They continually re-live things that are now gone, and their thoughts linger on how things were in the past. Life can be very difficult for people who are refugees, or displaced, or after wars, or when everyone they knew is dead.
Honeysuckle (Bach).
***

Past, unable to break from.

Too strongly influenced by exterior matters, inner self vulnerable, relies on opinions of others, fails to healthily adopt new structures which should replace the old ones as they fall away. Can be outdated in function and approach.
Walnut (Bach).
***

Peevish.
Forgets things, wherever he is he wants to be elsewhere. Some idiocy may be present.
Calc phos.
***

Peevish with homesickness and sleeplessness.
Capricious, looks for insults.
Caps.
***

Perfection, demands it of himself and everyone else.
Over-strict, unforgiving, inhuman, painful to have around. Hopeless bosses who antagonise everyone.
Rock water (Bach).
***

Perfection, standards too high.
Goes for the most demanding tasks, obsessive to control self and environment, tensions lead to leg and finger cramps.
Arsen alb.
***

Persecuted.
Sure he is being persecuted, deeply tired, hypochondria.
Plumb met.
***

Perseverance not there.

Fails to persevere in anything, tries this and tries that, goes here goes there, faints, wants sympathy, complains, mood switches.
Asaf.
***

Pessimistic.
People may program themselves into stages where they are only able to foresee negative outcomes. They seem unable to break this cycle of thought without help, even when logically it does not make sense. Hope vanishes. *Gorse (Bach).*
***

Petulant.
Senses injustice, caused by others, resentful, suppressed aggression, exaggerated blaming and seeking of scapegoats, avoids responsibility, acrid outbursts, not a good frame of mind for good focus.
Impatiens, Willow (all Bach).
***

Phobias (enduring fears, debilitating).
Phobias can severely curtail activities when energies are used to combat fear rather than to partake in life. To understand how a phobia can affect function, imagine feeling the terrors referred to in the following remedies, and then consider what it must be like to partake in life activities under those circumstances. Logic and explanations have no effect, as the problem is purely emotional.
Arguments or Western logic (Greek logic) cannot endure in the face of emotions. In our Western societies, which are completely subservient to emotion, yet overtly

completely run by logic, there will always be conflict. The subject cannot be discussed in depth in this book on homeopathy, which deals with remedies and their effect on emotions.

Claustrophobia is experienced by the person, and it may occur anywhere, feeling as if he were in a tunnel, or the dark is closing in, with events crushing him from all around, and he needs to escape the situation. *Stram.*

Storms fill the person with unimaginable terror, and madness seems at hand. *Rhod.*

Being alone fills the person with terrible fear. There is no protection, and vulnerability is traumatic. *Rad brom.*

Opposite sex encounters fill the sportsperson with nameless terrors. The terror is not experienced in groups of the same sex. *Puls.*

Irrational fears of spooks, or of illness, crowd the mind, destroying any chance of quiet focus on anything else. *Phos.*

Being responsible for anything brings great fear, and this type of person needs to avoid any sort of responsibility altogether. *Lyco.*

Water, or infection, both fill the mind with fears. *Hyos.*

The dark is viewed as filled with danger, terrifying. A person with this phobia cannot sleep in any dormitory, for instance, without keeping all the lights on. *Hydro ac, Caust.*

What may happen tomorrow, imagined in the seething fears feeding on themselves inside the head, bringing terror. *Calc carb.*

The touch of others brings huge dread. No contact sport can be entered into, nor can a masseur or doctor assist such people easily. *Brucea.*

Animal phobias fill the mind with fears, thinking of attacks, disease, and much more. Parades with animals in them must be avoided. *Bell.*

General anxiety, fear, anxiety about many imagined or impossible, or possible things in the future. A person consumed by imagined possibilities cannot compete effectively in life. *Arg nit.*

Births, and anticipated possible insanity, fill the mind with terrors. *Act race.*

Death is perceived as the most terrifying thing ever, disrupting any peace of mind and going round and round in the mind. *Acon.*

***

Plaintive speech.

Weepy, timid, makes mistakes, mutters, melancholic, forgets.

Crot horr.

***

Pleasure, gone.

Cannot enjoy or join in with activities around them, mentally weak and depleted, want to rest, no vital Force no power, unable to do sport.

Olive, Mustard (both Bach).

***

Plods on regardless.

This remedy is for when the will and courage to continue, has gone, when a breakdown seems imminent, when effort

and obstinate drive have reduced to despair. The remedy can restore strength and resilience.
Oak (Bach).
***

Poise, lack of.
Uncertain, cannot decide, too much input upsets him, very sensitive, neurosis, gait not purposeful.
Scleranthus (Bach).
***

Pouting.
Thinks others caused the problem, never sees own blame, resentment to minor faults of others, feels left out.
Willow, Chicory (both Bach).
***

Preaches at others.
Strongly identifies with values and principles, tries to control and influence others to be the same, self-justified, can be quite frantic, spiritual, cannot understand the views or personalities of other people.
Vervain, Rock water, Beech (all Bach).
***

Precise, dominating.
Obsessively exact and tidy, angry and violent, pompous, impulsive, craves respect.
Nux vom.
***

Pre-occupied.
Worrisome thoughts stuck inside, cannot be released, cyclical thinking patterns, no repose, not calm and serene. No concentration.
White chestnut (Bach).

***

Pride (unable to endure failure, critical of others).
Successful people need to be able to work towards goals,
enduring plenty of failure as they become more
accomplished. They need to be humble and able to analyse
why they have failed at any point, and also need to get on
amicably with other people, not criticizing them.
Lyco, Plat, Ver alb.
***

Procrastinates.
Weary mind does not react smoothly, tries to avoid action
or responsibility, is not focussed and clear, fuzzy thinking,
cannot get fully committed to activities or programs.
Hornbeam (Bach).
***

Public appearance, fear of.
Success nearly always demands some sort of public
appearance, hence the reason for some people's
desperation to do well, trying to find adulation. When a
person is filled with fear at the thought of a public
appearance, then good performance may be impossible.
One of the following remedies may very well remove this
fear, or diminish it to a lesser intensity
Gels, Arg nit, Lyco.
***

Quietness, longs for.
Far too excitable to relax quietly, confused, forgets things.
Sali ac.
***

R.
***

Rage.
Deep-seated raging anger, long-term, is best treated with
Staph, and short-term with *Bell,* and as a general easer of
turbulent emotions, the writer has had success with two
Damiana drops on the tongue daily, which will take a few
days to take effect. Rage can embitter and poison the body
and mind, lowering the immune system and wrecking
concentration. It may even cause the muscles to become
stiff and slow, spoiling physical activity.
Staph, Bell, Damiana drops.
***
Rage, apoplectic, sudden with pulsating blood flow.
Excitable, hypersensitive, pounding head.
Bella.
***
Rage, paroxysms.
Over-sexed, screaming insolence, violence possible.
Canth.
***
Rage uncontrolled.
Shortage of cognitive power, phobic reactions, ritualistic
patterns with shame attached, subconscious thoughts
surface, killing rages, destructive tempers.
Cherry plum (Bach) with Staph.
***
Reclusive.
May be evolved and educated, feels higher than others,
better bred, uneasy among friends, aloof, no camaraderie,
independent. Keeps away from group activities.
Water violet (Bach).
***

Red-faced rages.
Red cheeks, pulsing veins, hot hands and feet.
Sang canad.
***

Regression into the past.
Mourning that wonderful times cannot be repeated, homesick, empty-nest, dwells on the past instead of paying attention to what is happening, unable to focus on the present.
Honeysuckle (Bach).
***

Regrets.
Very aware of lost times and past happiness, never to be retrieved, powerless, empty, apathy, no life interest.
Honeysuckle, Pine (both Bach).
***

Relapses into old habits.
Cannot maintain concentration, just forgets now and repeats old habits, weak memory, no remorse, careless, reckless, cannot learn new skills, will not change with the times nor with training, unable to learn new skills etc.
Chestnut bud (Bach).
***

Release, longs for.
Strong conscience, community-minded, in tune with others, fearful and ambitionless people do community service as an escape, depressed at leaving own aspirations behind.
Centaury (Bach).
***

Religion, obsessive.

Feels entitled to control others, spiritual, strict path followed, real joy stifled at its roots but feigns religious joy, denial, ritualistic. Leads to physical cramps, rigidity, muscle disorders.
Rock water, Vervain (both Bach).
***

Remorse, filled with.
Burdened with guilt, broods with conscience, paranoia, longs for cleansing of the soul.
Pine (Bach).
***

Repressed spirit.
Restless, does not accept negatives as part of life itself, hates any disruption to inner self, alone, works for others instead of self, martyr, constant perceived setbacks put them down. Success is difficult to pursue while this attitude persists.
Agrimony, Centaury, Water violet (all Bach).
***

Resentment.
This may have the same effects as rage, becoming a long-term chronic disorder, leading to mental, emotional and physical illness. Deep-seated resentment interferes badly with living prowess.
Staph.
***

Resentment, chronic, growing.
Current things making one more and more resentful over time.
Holly, Willow (both Bach).
***

Resentful about petty politics.
Injustice, disgust, resentment, perspective may distort,
dissatisfaction, disillusionment.
Willow (Bach).
***

Reserved.
Haughty, lonely, refined, grown spiritually after hardships
in life, aloof, independent.
Water violet (Bach).
***

Resigned, gives up.
Confined inside self, not free in thought, stifled,
assertiveness gone, may be protecting self from life. Stale,
bored, unable to change, unmotivated. Accepts illness,
monotony, awful employment.
Wild rose, Centaury (both Bach).
***

Respect, deserves more.
Exuberance gone, apathy, not recognised for abilities,
avoids recreation, avoids engagement in group activities.
Water violet (Bach).
***

Responsibility makes him flustered.
Tasks seem insurmountable, discouraged, was joyful now
burdened, listless, cramps and fatigue from tension ruin
general ability.
Elm (Bach).
Runs away because he cannot face responsibilities.
Elm (Bach).
***

Restlessness, agitation, jumpiness, unbalanced.

Adjust your lifestyle, avoid long term tranquilizers. Your performance will suffer if you are not relaxed.

Hands and feet twitch and jerk, mind seems to remain in a frenzy of excitement. ***Tarent hisp.*** (St Vitus's dance)

Constant leg twitch and jerk. ***Meph puto.***

Constant rush, incoherent speech, strange and unrealistic opinions, need fresh air all the time. ***Lil tig.***

Taps rhythm incessantly, calmed by exercise, unable to keep still. ***Kali brom.***

Impulsive, thin, agitated, with a powerful need to eat and be cool, wants fresh air, hates noise, grumpy. ***Iod.***

Obsessively neat and perfect in everything, takes offence, impatient, greedy, never quiet or still. ***Arsen alb.***

***

Revenge.

Set on revenge, no matter the consequences or disruption. The entire system becomes poisoned with thoughts of revenge. Thoughts become, and remain circular.

Holly (Bach).

***

Romantic, overdoes it.

More into the idea than the reality, imagines wonderful things happening but does not see the real situation, unfulfilled, visions of great achievements and great things but they remain visions. Longing for death to re-unite with loved ones.

Clematis (Bach).

***

Routine bound.

Cannot stand people who interrupt normal routines.

Kali bich.

***

Routine, cannot stand it.
Fidgets, desperate for stimulation.
Calc phos.
***

Rushes all the time.
Never stops the flurry. Indigestion, wants alcohol to relax.
Sulph ac.
***

Rut, in.
Full of thoughts with too little action, feels hopeless, no
faith, cannot get into action.
Wild rose, Clematis, Gorse (all Bach).
***

Ruthless.
In his own mind he is the powerful leader, cruel,
insensitive, self-righteous, no forgiveness, anti-social.
Poorly accepted in the social situation.
Vine (Bach).
***

S.
***

Sadistic.
Sadistic people, and leaders, can stop proper development
in both character and physically, in those they can affect.
They have no understanding of how their behaviour
adversely affects their own cause.
Holly, Vine (both Bach).
***

Sadism with cruelty, callousness, mistrust.
Persecution complex, swears, no self-confidence.

Anac.
***
Sadness.
An all-pervading feeling that the world is so sad, that
everything has not gone the way it should have, that all is
lost, in spite of the potential it once had. It has been said
that Europe holds the biggest all-pervading feeling of
sadness ever felt. Sadness comes from disappointment,
alienation, anomie, not really coping with isolation.
Sadness affects one's entire life but can be treated
sometimes with remedies.
Lach.
***
Sanctimonious.
Feels superior to everyone, hypertension from suppression
of the feeling, heart and gastric problems, cannot stand
being disrespected, domineering, standards unrealistic,
critical, persecutory.
Rock water, Beech, Vervain, Vine (all Bach).
***
Sanity, doubts own.
Mind solid with unwanted impulses and urges, destructive
rage, terrible inner tensions use all energy, hyperactive,
oversensitive, sleep problems, all lead to poor life ability.
Cherry plum (Bach).
***
Satisfied, never.
Wants more and more, never happy with what he has, fear
of being ill forever, fear of medicines, afraid he will be
poisoned.
Allium sat.

***

Scathing comments.
Unstable interior results in threatening behaviour.
Emotions easily and suddenly incited, highly competitive,
abusive, low impulse control.
Holly, Beech (both Bach).
***

Sceptical, of everything.
Weak and unstable interior causes him to perceive
everything as threatening, causing sarcasm and vitriol,
seeks control of everything, no hopeful anticipation,
faultfinding, low compassion, hopeless team participant.
Beech, Vine, Gorse, Holly (all Bach).
***

Schizophrenia (see Nervous breakdown).
In spite of possible natural talents, or a desire to partake in
life, sufferers of schizophrenia are unlikely to be able to
participate. Their perceived worlds do not coincide with
the way it is necessary for the world to be seen, to take part
in it.
These people live in their own world, out of contact with
this world. Sometimes they have a split personality, and
are two different people. They are usually unable to care
for themselves.
Mind and body seem split, with contradictory demands, so
person is confused and angry. ***Anac.***
Think they are two people, one part of body is detached
from the rest, feel unable to be healed. ***Bapt.***
Sudden mood swings, euphoria, fear of insanity, delusions
of grandeur, possibly in contact with supranatural powers
and beings. ***Cann indic.***

Hallucinations, amazing imaginings, possible bi-polar disorder, possibly violent. They should be watched for mania, are very energetic, can be filled with religious fervour. ***Stram.***
***

School phobia.
This phobia, in itself, may not interfere with life too much, apart from school. However, it is very possibly a symptom of much further reaching problems than are immediately apparent. These other problems may cause major disruptions of life activities.
This can be a very complicated situation to deal with. It is erroneously viewed as a disorder most of the time, although, while it can be, it may not be at all. It could be caused by claustrophobia, so see that section in this book. It may be something that can be attended to by using the section on fears. It could be homesickness, so try that section. There may be certain phobias, so you need to look at that section. The teacher is likely to be "closed-minded" (sees only one solution per problem and can only see the official way of seeing things), while the child may be "open-minded", questioning irrelevant or pointless aspects of schooling. The child may not be able to respond in the formal way by using words, so therefore is judged a dunce. Disorders like dyslexia may prevent the child from responding in the conventional way, even though he could be highly intelligent, and therefore he is labelled a dunce. The child's social background may be very different from the teacher's, or even other pupils, so a real connection or understanding is never achieved. In some cases, teachers simply take a hate towards particular children, and keep

them back, making their lives a hell on earth. There is a phenomenon called the "self-fulfilling prophecy", whereby a pupil may only ever achieve to where a teacher decides he will achieve. Certain schools have no discipline, allowing disruptive and chaotic behaviour, cheeking teachers, and other sad behaviour patterns. The child may suffer from ADHD, or perhaps agoraphobia. Parents who failed to achieve, may pressure their children beyond endurance, while others may constantly mock the system, so destroying any respect for it, in the child's mind. Poverty or drug-dependence at home may make the child feel obliged to be out working, rather than at school. Huge families may make a child feel obliged to stay at home to look after babies. Single-parent families may pressure the child to baby-sit while the parent works. Melancholia may be working its evils in the child's mind.

This is only the tip of the iceberg, but the point is that a really good look at the entire situation, by a well-qualified person, is often essential. A person from within the system can only see the situation from the conventional point of view, and may try to preserve the status quo by carefully avoiding the real problems. Until society evolves to a point where children are not imprisoned and coerced into 12 or 13 years of forced-labour, sometimes under conditions utterly intolerable to some children, we will be faced with school phobia, and much worse.

It is no co-incidence that certain countries have massive child-suicide rates, and massive illegitimacy rates among schoolchildren, and enormous depression problems, coupled with unbelievable bullying. They, like school phobia, are all symptoms of a deep underlying sickness in the society, which cannot be cured by simply administering pills to individual children.

How then, do you cope when your child has school phobia? Remember that it only lasts a while before the child leaves school, so try a holding exercise initially, in conjunction with a therapist, a homeopath and possibly a psychologist not employed by the system. Try to put yourself in the child's place, alienated and anomic in school, desperately unhappy, becoming physically ill, perhaps bullied, no place to go, and that means no-one to turn to who will really help. Then weigh up the possibilities of moving schools, moving countries, home-schooling, private schooling, or leaving school as soon as possible. It may be better to leave sooner rather than later, before your child commits suicide, or is scarred for life.

***

Scorned, feels scorned and mortified.
Honour lost, wounded, grief, anger, disappointed, self-righteous, failed love, muscle cramps, missionaries sometimes, trying to convert others to their ideas.
Ver alb.
***

Screaming in fear.
Gnaws fists and nails, wants to die, terrible forebodings, suddenly laughs and sings.
Acon.
***

Scruffy.
Feels no hope ahead, drive and anticipation come to a stop, low Vital Force, giving up, weak mind prevents him from

coping with normal matters, erratic behaviour, work declines.
Wild rose, Hornbeam, Gorse (all Bach).
***

Secretive.
Delusional, threatened, paranoid sometimes, emotions rapidly aroused, vengeful, plotting, ulcers, thwarted ambition, rages, generally physically disordered, unable to be dedicated in life tasks.
Holly (Bach).
***

Security in relationships craved.
Always trying to make a solid social structure for himself. Failure leads to spleen and liver disorders.
Arsen alb.
***

Self-confidence lacking.
Certain to fail because he thinks he will. Feels others are always better. Stands down.
Larch (Bach).
***

Self-esteem undermined.
Threatened feeling, poor self-image possible, seeks recognition, peace-loving, has a feeling of inferiority somewhere, anger at being disregarded.
Lyco.
***

Self-image, awful.
Ashamed of self, feels dirty, compulsive washer and cleaner, imagines personal flaws are terrible, despair, feels persecuted, skin diseases, fear of infections, guilt, broods,

seeks perfection in all he does, ritual-bound, cannot relax and enjoy life.
Crab apple, Pine (both Bach).
***

Self-opinionated.
Cannot be contradicted, must control everyone, tense and stiff, migraines, tries to dominate others, no empathy, always right, disruptive, poor manners, arrogant, gastric ulcers, hypertension from suppression of hate and enmity, useless as a team participant, cannot be taught, always knows better.
Vine, Vervain, Beech, Chicory, Impatiens (all Bach).
***

Self-pity.
Unable to grasp that affairs are caused by himself, always blames others, mighty inner resentment, disorders caused by having to suppress aggression towards others, looks for scapegoat, sense of failure, histrionics, overly activated mannerisms, tight and rigid, needs to change attitude before he can do well in anything.
Willow, Chicory (both Bach).
***

Self-reproach.
Conscience too active, burdened, cannot release despondency and recover, stifles inside own mind, ritualistic, deep guilt, remorse, violent rages, heart, lung and digestive disorders result from the mental disorder, sport declines steadily.
Pine (Bach).
***

Self-reproach with persecution.

Dull and morose, sadness and happiness alternating, hallucinations of two other people in her bed, imaginary grief and imagining she is alone and persecuted.
Cyclamen.
***

Self-righteous.
Willful, dominant, possessive, opinionated.
Dulc.
***

Self-sacrificial.
Overcare for others to the detriment of the self, tries to control others, disciplined and routined, set jaw type of person, addicted to self-mastery, joyless, emotionally stagnant, no fun to have in a team.
Rock water (Bach).
***

Self-trust, gone.
Despondent, dreads performing, intimidated, hesitant, may show off in response, low drive and stamina, low immune system, not self-reliant, analyses self, shy, tries to identify with others, may feel he is two people, poor in group activities.
Larch, Cerato (both Bach).
***

Senses depressed.
Acuity of senses lost, taciturn, sad, slurred words, sighs, apprehension, thoughts with no clarity. Muscle control poor.
Hell nig.
***

Sensitive, too quick to react, angry, impatient.

From alcohol, overwork, vertigo, hay fever, sour stomach with eructations, paroxysmal coughs, hot skin but feels cold.
Nux vom.
***

Sequence and order obsession.

Collectors, sexual obsessions, wringing hands, highly agitated, aggressive, very jealous, may injure themselves.
Hyosc nig.
***

Serious, takes life too seriously.

Everything seen as important and serious, cannot even contemplate failure.
Aurum met.
Takes on too much, works to collapse.
Calc carb.
Sense of duty too strong, with mindless adherence to rules, stress leads to heart attacks.
Kali carb.
Compulsive, obsessive drive for detail and perfection, full of fears with no reason.
Arsen alb.
***

Servile.

Over-concerned about how others might react, exploited by others, suppresses own potential and becomes ill as a result, overcompliant, broods over own failings, no pride, nightmares and insomnia, no drive to overcome obstacles in life.
Centaury, Agrimony, Pine (all Bach).
***

Setback, caused by something specific.
Discouraged, sad, weakened, drive diminished by
something known.
Gentian (Bach).
***

Severe, inhuman.
Obsessively tries to control others, self-martyrdom, joy
destroyed in the very soul of the person, denial, discipline,
numbness.
Rock water, Vine (both Bach).
***

Shame, deep.
Guilt, conscience, suicidal, despair, always blames
circumstances or others, grinds teeth, hates self, secretive,
cleans everything ritualistically. Poor focus.
Crab apple, Pine (both Bach).
***

Shiftless, lazy.
Ducks and dives, avoids work, hypochondriacal, too many
interests and too little focus, self-centred, philosopher,
possible intellectual.
Sulph.
***

Shock or trauma (see Bereavement, Grief).
Blood pressure may drop, blood supply to organs drops,
resulting in tiredness, apathy, coldness, blue colour,
nausea, thirst, faintness, shallow breathing, anxiety,
confusion possible.
The other result of shock may be the inability of the heart
to pump adequately, similar to heart attacks, cerebral

trauma or haemorrhage, kidney failure, poisoning, infection, or fright.

Stop any bleeding possible and clear the airways, get the patient breathing, lay them flat to allow blood supply to the entire body, turning the head on its side, loosening any tight clothing. Cover them lightly but do not allow any drinking of fluids or eating. Treat with homeopathic remedies while awaiting an ambulance. Do not take shock lightly as it is potentially lethal.

Arn, China, Acon, Arsen, Carbo veg, Rescue Remedy.
Sometimes the upper body is hot and the lower body is cold.

For fainting and vertigo with eyes sunken in, falling down. ***Acet ac.***

After any great shock or fear of death, cannot relax, faints when rising up. ***Acon.***

Blue, exhausted, stupified, diarrhoea, weak, poor breathing and heartbeat. ***Camph.***

Rolling about with spasms and cramps, gasping occasionally. ***Cup met.***

Cardiac shock, heart attack, faint and weak, bluish, eyes dilated. ***Digit.***

After the shock, pain in the heart, feeling of suffocation, rips clothing off chest or throat, gasps and sighs, non-stop talking. ***Lach.***

***

Shows off, noisily.

Inappropriate reaction to environment, shies away from discord, restless and needing peace inside, covers up inner turmoil by showing off, inner torture, insensitive to the reactions of others and so unable to lead well but feels like

a born leader, disruptive, anti-social, bad for any team or group.
Vine, Agrimony (both Bach).
***
Shy.
Fearful, anticipates unpleasantness, intimidated, fears making things worse, does not want to be seen or watched, passive, no good for activities in a social setting.
Mimulus (Bach), Lyco.
Extreme shyness with fear of situations. *Baryta carb.*
***
Sleep disorders (see Insomnia).
A tired person does not recover quickly nor properly from activities. Immune systems also become weakened, with consequent illnesses, colds and flu's. Cut out all stimulants, especially caffeine and cigarettes. Eliminate all disturbing or adrenaline-creating pastimes, habits and activities, entertainments.
Attend to diet, relaxation and exercise. Take up meditation or yoga.
Tiredness after a meal, need a nap, grumpy. *Nux vom.*
Sleepy after eating but a nap causes irritability. *Lyco.*
Episodes of sleepiness during the day. *Opium.*
Depressed person, sleeps after meals and bloats up. *Nux mosch.*
Wanders around at night, has no recollection next day.
Kali brom, Stram.
***
Sleep disorders, intermittent, from internal conflicts.
Agrimony (Bach).
Hostility keeps emerging, not resolved. *Willow (Bach).*

Fears surrounding inner conflicts. ***Mimulus (Bach).***
For thoughts causing escalating fears and tension. ***Cherry plum (Bach).***
Same thoughts and emotions constantly recur and keep one awake. ***White chestnut (Bach).***
Agitated thinking patterns disturb sleep. ***Vervain (Bach).***
***

Slow, feels slow and too big.

Feels hurried but feels as if he is moving so slowly, time is so slow, feels so heavy, everything seems unreal, sneering, and suicidal if he sees a knife.

Alumina.
***

Slow thinking.

Unreliable thinking process, dim-witted (unusual for this person), lack of interest in everyday matters, closed-minded.

Carbo veg.
***

Sluggish and fat.

Slow in everything, may tend to obesity.

Carbo veg.
***

Smoking, after effects.

Loses control of the mind after smoking, headaches, confusion associated with cigarettes. Feels poisoned by cigarettes.

Calad seg.
***

Snobbish.

Loneliness, self-chosen isolation because of a feeling of superiority, urgent need to drill any listener without offering them any chance to speak, wishes to be understood, talks too much, tells everyone of illness, fixations, full of pride, deep anger. Spoils groups and camaraderie.
Rock water, Beech, Vine, Heather, Chicory (all Bach).
***

Solitude (craves for).
This may be useful for sportspeople such as fishermen, or even long-distance runners, but is detrimental for such activities as rugby, or others where other people are present.
Sep.
***

Someone behind.
Sensation of a person behind him all the time, changing emotions, alone, stares, does not tidy house.
Brom.
***

Spaced out.
Not interested in the present, reveries and imaginings, unable to get into action, absent-minded, mind-body disconnection with lethargy, poor memory, clairvoyant, cannot get into life effectively.
Clematis (Bach).
***

Speaking trouble, no idea what to say.
Feels dull and slow, anxious, weary.
Merc.
***

Spinning room, hammering in head.
May experience terror of solitude and horror of work.
Cad sulph.
***

Spiteful.
Vexed, acrimonious, negative, shows hatred, anger and jealousy, intolerance, a weak person inside, disliked in teams or groups.
Holly (Bach).
***

Spiteful but hard-working.
Anxious about health, agitated, thumping heart, fastidious.
Arsen alb.
***

Squeamish.
Over-careful of things, tries to stop bad things happening, shy, timid, fears, may exhibit bravado to conceal squeamishness.
Mimulus, Crab apple (both Bach).
***

Stagnated.
Mind preoccupied or diverted, thinks of past rather than future, nostalgia rather then forward planning, low Vital Force, absent from the present, negative expectancy may be present, flat expression, psychotic sometimes, cannot progress in life.
Wild rose, Honeysuckle, Gorse, Mustard (all Bach).
***

Stamina, emotional, none.

Dreams long submerged, vital urges gone, expects nothing good, emaciated, discouraged, creativity gone, no goals, no further interest in life.
Centaury, Gorse, Gentian, Olive, Hornbeam, Clematis, Wild rose (all Bach).
***

Stifled enjoyment.
Unable to relax and enjoy, stifles emotions, perhaps disappointed in life, or beset with grief that will not leave.
Nat mur.
***

Stifled people becoming introverted.
Capacity never expressed or used, becoming fixed in ideas and impulses, with shame they injure themselves.
Sil.
***

Strangers, afraid of.
Fearful of any possible bad things, fear of real things not imaginary, nervous, timid, inner fears. A problem for social encounters.
Mimulus, Holly (both Bach).
***

Struggle unending.
Sees life, and work, as a perpetual, long, never-ending battle, with no time to recuperate or think, or to enjoy and relax.
Oak plus Olive plus Agrimony (all Bach).
***

Storms (fear of).
Fear is debilitating. It is also not logical, so cannot be talked away easily. For someone who lives in a stormy

area, this can cause huge disruption to life. A storm the night before, can leave a person exhausted and lifeless the next day.

Rhod, Nat mur, Acon.
***

Stubborn.

Feels superior and justified in all own ideas and judgements, intolerant of other people's ideas and views, fixations of criticism to specific others, paranoid personality disorder. Mentally and physically rigid and unbending, poor team people.

Vervain, Vine, Chicory, Beech (all Bach).
***

Stubborn and angry.

Bores nose, picks at skin, bleeds.

Arum triph.
***

Stupidity, intolerant of.

Rigid, intolerant, never wrong, irritable but feels fully justified, lonely, hates delays, driven, tense and tight and not good at teamwork.

Beech, Vine, Impatiens (all Bach).
***

Stupified.

Fears, angers, griefs, disturbances, hysteria, feels hollow, empty, tremors and cramps, spasms, falls down.

Cocc indic.
***

Stupor.

Dull, slow, indifferent, sighs, sleepless, restless.

Ailan gland.

***

Subservient.
Subjugates own interests, avoids upsetting anyone, dependent personality disorder, is exploited by others, no drive in life.
Centaury (Bach).
***

Suffocating from people or talking.
Hurtful comments result, poor control, suffocates, unable to breathe properly, spasm of glottis.
China.
***

Suicidal anguish.
Hopeless, disgust with life, rages at any contradiction, brooding melancholy, morose, weeps, prays, talks too much, vexed, asks streams of questions and waits for no answers, hysteria, quarrelsome, feels he has neglected his duties.
Aur met.
***

Suicidal to escape everything.
Lives in reveries so never fulfilled, sleepless, thoughts vanish, forgets things, clairvoyant, sees suicide as an escape from a pointless existence.
Clematis, Agrimony (both Bach).
***

Suicidal.
Sport may help to keep these impulses at bay, but if suicide has become a focal point, then it will detract from sporting ability.
Blood, knives, cutting meat, may trigger suicide. *Alum.*

Uncontrollable (almost) impulses, such as suicide may be controlled sometimes. ***Aur met.***
Sudden suicidal impulses, possibly after meals, storms or alcohol, can possibly be controlled. ***Naja.***
Sick of life, wants to end everything. ***Nat sulph.***
***

Sulking.
An introverted sulker may experience difficulties taking part in sport, especially group sports or group activities. Refuses to speak to others. ***Sep.***
Introverted, wants solitude, brooding. ***Nat mur.***
Prolonged sulking. ***Ign.***
***

Superstition, evil, ghosts.
Superstitions about murder and death, anxiety.
Rhus tox.
***

Suppression of anger and annoyance.
Has to be too kind and helpful, cannot show rebellion, emotional tensions lead to illness.
Impatiens (Bach).
***

Suppression of powerful, vital impulses.
Must appear compliant and gentle, outwardly.
Agrimony.
***

Suspicious (of everyone, everything).
Remember that suspicion and alertness to others and the environs, has kept many people alive over the centuries. What you see here may sometimes be a leftover from millions of years back, a survival mechanism which

worked very well. Sometimes therapy is required to calm
it, and sometimes a remedy may help. Too much suspicion
takes the mind and focus off everything else.

Anac.

Holly (Bach).
***

Switches of emotion.

Heavy, deep sighs, yawns, changes of sensation, laughs
then cries, loves then hates, rages and repents.

Croc sat.
***

Sympathy, craves.

Overdoes things to get sympathy, or may passively make
themselves seen to attract sympathy, ulterior motives in
actions, helpfulness designed to attract sympathy,
manipulates people where possible, feigns troubles or
illness for attention. Wants to be understood and
supported, feels injustice in the mind, seethes with inner
angers sometimes, at his lot.

Chicory, Heather, Willow (all Bach).
***

T.
***

Tactless.

Insensitive so can never lead well, but imagine they are
born leaders, can be abusive, ambitious, strong willpower
and very self-righteous, arrogant, egotistic, do not co-
operate, try to intimidate, suffer from hypertension and
gastric ulcers.

Vine, Chicory, Impatiens, Beech, Vervain (all Bach).
***

Tantrums in children and adults (see Temper).
This phenomenon may arise from various causes, including incomplete development, immaturity, poor self-discipline, lack of discipline in the home, school and society, poor social integration, alienation from society, emotional or psychological disorders. Tranquillizers and sedatives may mask the underlying problem and leave it in place. Psychological and homeopathic treatment may help remove the real problems. Jail may make it worse, but is an option used by society, to protect people from those who have tantrums.

Tempers may be moderated and become manageable when people immerse themselves in sport, burning off frustrations with hard exercise, but this is not always the case. Tempers may prevent people from being welcome in team events, or cause poor behaviour in the gym, dojo, or whatever.

Tantrums are the adult equivalent of a naughty child which throws itself to the floor and screams blue murder.

For restless, bad tempered children. ***Cham.***

For overworked, profane adults. ***Anac.***

For overbearing, overactive, explosive adults. ***Nux vom.***

Tantrums, accompanied by neuralgic pains, spasms and cramps. ***Coloc.***

Suppressed temper with stomach cramps and urinary problems, hypersensitive adults. ***Staph.***
***

Task too huge, dreams recede.
Dream is clear, in sight, real, but the task seems too big, vacillates, procrastinates, fearful of doing what is required. ***Germ.***

***

Tearful, crying.
Sighing and crying. *Ign.*
On the verge of tears permanently. *Nat mur.*
Cries for no reason, wants company. *Puls.*
Cries for no reason, avoids company, gets much worse when consoled. *Sep.*
***

Tears, suddenly, unexpectedly.
Restless, suicidal, no sensual enjoyment, fear of poisoning, dreams of exercise.
Rhus tox.
***

Tearfully sentimental.
From the very depths of the person, too strongly influenced by external factors, unable to evaluate effectively, not quite able to discern the real value of ideas, admires others and emulates them, deep marks left by unwholesome events, fragile, mind not anchored in the present, happiness and the past seems lost forever, poor focus.
Honeysuckle, Walnut (both Bach).
***

Tedium, too much.
Mind not sharpened, poor concentration, judgement weakens, dreams die inside, seeks seclusion, leaves sport.
Clematis, Hornbeam, Wild rose (all Bach).
***

Temper, sudden and hot.
Red-faced outbursts, vertigo, coldness follows with faintness and trembling of the arms possible.
Sulph.

***

Tentative.

Too careful, fearful, scared of life matters not imaginings, low confidence, fear of failure, intimidated, no drive and courage.

Mimulus, Larch, Cerato, Scleranthus (all Bach).
***

Terrors (night) (see Panic, Fear).

Night terrors can leave a person debilitated and exhausted, mentally and physically, and in no state to do much.

Kali brom, Stram.

Children with nightmares and night terrors. *Hyosc, Stram.*

Fidgety children with worms and terrors. *Cina.*

Grinding of teeth, moaning and groaning. *Kali brom.*

Terror free-floating, sense of foreboding, no reason.

Aspen, Rock rose (both Bach).

Catching fear from others. *Rock rose (Bach).*
***

Theatrical.

Shies from discord, pretends all is well, acts theatrically to show how well all is although it's not well, blames others, resentful, no forgiveness.

Agrimony, Willow (both Bach).
***

Thick-skinned.

Insensitive, imagines he is very powerful, no-one will follow him, refuses to co-operate, stressed, poor team player and unpleasant as an opponent or partner.

Vine (Bach).
***

Thinking unclear, ineffective.

Moans, complains.
Mag phos.
***

Thinking very difficult, apathetic, lazy.
Headache and vomitting, nose, skin and stomach troubles,
pains and illness all over. *Sulph.*
***

Thoughts, of past.
Fails to lock mind onto the present, unresolved matters of
the past disturb life focus needed in the present.
Honeysuckle (Bach).
***

Thunder (terror) (see Storms).
This may stem from past events, but is very real and
exhausting for the sufferer.
Gels.
***

Thwarted, constantly.
Feels lonely, does not work together with others to achieve
goals, agitated and on edge, abides by fixed principles, can
go manic or catatonic, weak interior, not an effective and
relaxed group participant.
Vervain, Impatiens, Beech, Walnut (all Bach).
***

Tics.
Minor tics should pose no problem for most people and the
tics may not be noticed. However, serious jerks could
perhaps detract from the social side of life, or the
communicating side.
Thuja, Arg nit, Lyco.
***

Ties, old ties too strong.
Friends or family from the past still exert a hold which is
over-strong, and which hinders and restricts going ahead
mentally and emotionally.
Walnut (Bach).
***

Tight clothing, aversion to, talks non-stop.
Septic blood, infections, gangrene, dislikes warmth,
symptoms move from the left to the right side of the body,
suffocating coughs, worse when waking up, lump in throat,
fevers.
Lach.
***

Time, no conception.
Misjudges and miscalculates, always late for projects,
work and arrangements, miscalculates time required, loses
sense of the right time, seems unreliable, not anchored in
the real present, cannot be relied on to keep to schedules
and be ready for meetings etc.
Clematis, Wild rose (both Bach).
***

Timid and slow, superstitious.
Fears being alone, slow to understand things, lazy, does
pointless things, no interest nor perseverance.
Con mac.
***

Tired, with life.
Despondent, insurmountable problems imagined, desolate,
anguish, fails to see any advantage, suicidal, no salvation
seen, normal activities impossible.
Sweet chestnut (Bach).

***
Tolerance, none.
Only own views countenanced, no other views or opinions even considered, vicious, sarcastic, antagonistic, can do no wrong in own eyes, thinks self is all-powerful and intelligent, cannot accept teaching or instruction, a hopeless team participant and hopeless leader.
Beech, Chicory, Vine, Vervain, Impatiens (all Bach).
***
Touchy, ugly, dissatisfied.
May feel they are evil. Uneasy. Children will not be carried or stroked.
Cina.
***
Touch, aversion to.
This would preclude sufferers from engaging in contact sports.
Arn.
Piercing pain when touched. ***Bry.***
Pain eased by touch. ***Rhus tox.***
After shock, constantly insists nothing is wrong when clearly there is plenty wrong. ***Arn.***
Dying people sometimes scream at people who try to touch them to help them, and may even attack them.
***
Touch, fear of.
Bed too hard to sleep, angry, fearful, rage followed by tears, insists he is well, thoughts escape him, delirium, muttering, feels worthless, gets frights, thinks deeply.
Arnica.
***

Tongue-tied.
No faith in own opinions at all, timid, fears upsetting anyone, avoids any possible confrontation, avoids people.
Mimulus, Larch (both Bach).
***

Trapped, stagnated, unable to get going.
Worried, stuck, must go forward but seem glued to the spot.
Graph, Germ.
***

Trembles with fear needs to urinate.
Lots of fears, especially falling from a height, or heart stopping. Feels inadequate to the occasion and life.
Gels.
***

Trivialities assume huge proportions.
Clumsy, rushed, hard done by, wants attention then spurns it.
Nat mur.
***

Trivialities obsess the mind.
Temper, irritability, manic, restless, on edge, nervous breakdown possible, fails to see the bigger picture, rigid focus, feels flawed and not good-looking.
Crab apple, Impatiens, Beech (all Bach).
***

Trust absent.
Unable to trust, suspicious of others, vexed, greedy.
Holly (Bach).
***

Turbulence of the mind.

Desires peace, suppresses conflict (which emerges in other forms), intolerant to disharmony or interruption, reacts too much to external stimuli, no mental peace, hysterical neurosis, cannot concentrate on anything in mental peace.
Agrimony, White chestnut, Scleranthus (all Bach).
***

Turmoil of emotions.
Wants to live and wants to die, confused and gloomy, worse when spoken to, anxious.
Nat sulph.
***

Two selves, near death.
Convinced there are two of him and he is dying.
Petrol.
***

U.
***

Ugly behaviour, dread.
Irritable, sure home is not home and wants to go elsewhere, wants things then throws them away, fear and dread of the future.
Bry.
***

Ugly, thinks one is.
Self-disgust, shame about looks, feels dirty and cleans all the time, feels rejected, too ashamed to succeed in anything.
Crab apple (Bach).
***

Unappreciated, not valued:

Antagonistic to anyone who disagrees with him, thinks fate is against him, talents not recognised.
Calc sul.
***

Understanding of events poor.
Seems not to comprehend anything going on, no interest in people or surroundings.
Phos ac.
***

Uneasy, all the time.
Deep uneasiness, rituals offer some protection, ghosts and spirits threaten, phobias of all sorts.
Aspen (Bach).
***

Unfettered by conventions.
Goes to extremes for satisfaction, larger than life, normal life too humdrum and boring, needs far more stimulation than most people do, always unfulfilled, the condition can assist or impede general life ability.
Wild oat, Clematis (both Bach).
***

Unhappiness, no reason, just a cloud descending.
This may perhaps be caused by chemical changes, or by matters not in the conscious mind. It may come and go without warning. *Mustard (Bach).*
***

Unreasonable.
Thwarted ambitions, domineering posture, overbearing attitude, gastric ulcers, hypertension and much more, unco-operative, tensed up, lonely, uncontrolled anger leading to

jarring and unacceptable attitude, feels superior to
everyone else, impossible to have in a group or team.
Vine, Beech, Impatiens (all Bach).
***

Unreliable, lacks courage, not a stable person.
Unhelpful, weak, cannot take strain or persevere, no inner
strength., hides exhaustion.
Oak (Bach).
***

Unresponsive.
Life requires alertness and rapid response, to any changes.
A drop in response ability probably requires treatment.
Deep emotional problems, tearful sighing. ***Act race.***
A long period of worry leaves emotional deadness. ***Ambra
gris.***
Unstable, moody, self-centred women. ***Cocc.***
Huge disruptive setbacks have taken place in life. ***Ign.***
After a tragedy, excited in the morning but completely
unresponsive at night. ***Lach.***
Alternating ebullience and apathy. ***Nux mosch.***
Laughing and crying all the time, women who are fearful
of men. ***Puls.***
Moan and groan, do nothing, undergoing explosive
changes from apathy, to agitation and excitement. ***Ver alb.***
Unresponsive, indecisive, not alert.
Graph.
***

Unsuccessful after long efforts.
Disappointment and deep grief, cannot wait longer to
achieve, spasms and contractions.
Ign.

***

Unsettled, cannot settle down to tasks and life.
Constantly fretting and restless, cannot see ordinary tasks
through, never content.
Agrimony (Bach).
***

V.
***

Vacant.
No concentration, no interest, indifferent, bemused, not
there, withdrawn.
Clematis (Bach).
***

Vacilatory.
Torn between possibilities, cannot decide, uncertain.
Scleranthus (Bach).
***

Vengeful.
Deterred in their intentions by outer influences, defensive,
aggressive, vexed, envious, competitive, imagines honour
is undermined, wrong attitude for group interaction, and
unsuitable for team activities.
Holly (Bach).
***

Vertigo (see Dizziness).
This can be a drawback for those who would like to do
bungee-jumping or parachuting, or rock-climbing, or pot-
holing.
Heights, fear of. *Arg nit, Hyper.*
At anytime or place, fear of heights. *Con mac.*
***

Vexed, ugly behaviour.
Uncivil, children must be carried, want things then reject
them, piteous moaning and complaining, impatient,
intolerant, spiteful.
Cham.
***

Victimised, feels.
Feels others obstruct all intentions and aims, aggressive
attitude encourages others to obstruct him, plotting and
vengeful, hatred and jealousy, tenseness, violent subconscious urges, bad in a team, poor social attitude.
Cherry plum, Holly (both Bach).
***

Victimised, resentful.
Deep hates, anger, oversensitive yet will not defend own
interests, subdued, never achieves because he does not go
out and do things, self-righteously overdoes care for others,
ulterior motives in actions, histrionic personality disorder.
Willow, Chicory, Centaury, Mimulus (all Bach).
***

Vulnerable, threatened.
Feels threatened from things which cannot possibly
threaten him in any way at all, such as a car that went past,
angry and defensive.
Arnica.
***

W.
***

Walks great distances.
Strong impulse to travel far by foot.
Bursa past.

***
Weeps, for no reason.
Will not be consoled, fears he is incurably ill, gets frights, sad, thinks something bad will happen, taciturn alternating with cheerfulness.
Cact grand.
****
Weepy, clingy, whiney people.
Needs constant comforting, discharge from eyes and nose, blocked ears, indigestion, dry throat, upset stomach, short of breath, itching. *Puls.*
***
Welfare of others a constant worry.
Continuously frets about whether other people are safe and well, pre-occupied, apprehensive, constantly upset by trifles.
But ac., Zinc sul.
***
Wild, irrational ideas and uncontrolled thoughts.
Cherry plum (Bach).
***
Will subjugated.
Weak, a doormat, never says no, intimidated, servile.
Centaury (Bach).
***
Winning.
Any obsession can be seen as a disorder of the mind, especially if losing makes the person angry and ill, with long term after-effects.
This remedy is for someone who always has to be the best, who wants to be the leader, who works tirelessly to do

everything perfectly, so as to receive admiration from others, and when these goals are not achieved, illness follows. The person is very responsible, hard-working, dedicated, efficient, community-minded, but only to achieve personal goals. There is reliability and strength, visible to others, but a desperate need to have the admiration of others too. Great anger may surface when admiration is not forthcoming, with self-doubt, anxiety and loss of confidence. Aur met.

The person discussed above may be very sensitive, easily hurt, offended, disappointed and humiliated, full of rage but not showing the anger. So instead, other people are "punished" by hypochondria appearing, with imaginary critical heart diseases, fatal disorders, designed to teach a lesson to the indifferent others around. Very low esteem comes about when others may not notice, with deep melancholy and even possible suicide. Treatment for this condition, *Aur met.*
***

Worry (deep, work, money, exhaustion).
Life is completely disrupted by deep, undermining worries.
Kali brom.
Huge, fearsome worries, senses injustice, digestive system seriously in disorder.
Caust.
***

Wrong, everything.
Foolish and silly, cannot focus for any time, weeps and complains, mania then indifference, hysteria, groundless fears.
Apis mel.

***

Y.

***

Yielding.

Stands back, gives way, needs protection, needs affection, needs shelter, obliging, no drive nor strong emotion.

Puls.

***

Z.

***

Zombie.

Lives in day-dreams and reveries, not capable of pinning down thoughts and actions, longs for release from life, vertigo, spaced out, has no drive.

Clematis (Bach).

***

35. Remedies and frequent abbreviations.
***

A.
***

Abro: Abrotanum
Absinth: Absinthium
Acet ac: Acetic acid
Acon: Aconitum napellus
Act race: Act(a)ea racemosa
Aesc hips: Aesculus hippocastanum
Aeth: Aethusa cynapium
Agar (musc): Agaricus muscarius-amanita
Agnus castus: Agnus castus
Agrimony: Bach Flower Remedy
Ailan gland: Ailanthus glandulosa
Allium sat: Allium sativum (garlic)
Aloe: Aloe
Alum: Alumina
Ambra gris: Ambra grisea (whale)
Amm carb: Ammonium carb
Amm mur: Ammonium muriaticum
Anac orient: Anacardium orientalis
Ant crud: Antimonium crudum
Antipyrine: Antipyrene
Apis mel: Apis mellifica
Arg met: Argentum metallicum
Arg nit: Argentum nitricum
Arn: Arnica
Ars alb: Arsenicum album
Arum triph: Arum triphyllum

Asaf: Asafoetida
Asarum europ: Asarum europum
Aspen: Bach Flower Remedy
Aur fluor: Aurum fluoricum
Aur (met): Aurum metallicum
Aur nit: Aurum nitricum
Aur sul mag: Aurum sulphuratum
***

B.
***

Bap(tista): Baptista
Baryta c: Baryta carbonate
Beech: Bach Flower Remedy
Bell: Belladonna
Berb: Berberis vulgaris
Bismuth: Bismuthum
Bov: Bovista
Brom: Bromum
Brucea: Brucea
Bry: Bryonia
Bufo: Bufo (toad)
Bursa past: Bursa pastoris
But ac: Butyric acid (butter)
***

C.
***

Cact: Cactus grandiflorus
Cad met: Cadmium metallicum
Cad sulph: Cadmium sulphuricum
Cal seg: Caladium seguinum (arum)
Calc carb: Calcarea carbonica

Calc fluor: Calcarea fluorica
Calc phos: Calcarea phosphorica
Calc sulph: Calcarea sulphurica
Calend: Calendula officinalis
Cann indic: Cannabis indica
Cann sat: Cannabis sativa
Canth: Cantharis
Caps an: Capsicum annuum
Carbo veg: Carbo vegetabilis
Carcin: Carcinosin
Causticum: Causticum
Centaury: Bach Flower Remedy
Cerato: Bach Flower Remedy
Cer ceps: Cereus ceps
Cham: Chamomilla
Chel: Chelidonium majus
Cherry plum: Bach Flower Remedy
Chestnut bud: Bach Flower Remedy
Chicory: Bach Flower Remedy
China: Cinchona officinalis
Cic: Cicuta virosa
Cimi: Cimifuga racemosa
Cina: Cina (Worm seed)
Clematis: Bach Flower Remedy
Clem erec: Clematis erecta
Coca: Cocaina
Cocc indic: Cocculus indicus
Coff (crud): Coffea cruda
Colch aut: Colchicum autumnalis (Saffron)
Coloc: Colocynthis
Con mac: Conium maculata (Hemlock)

Crab apple: Bach Flower Remedy
Crocus: Crocus sativa
Crot (hor): Crotalis horridus
Cyc or Cycl: Cyclamen
***

D.
***

Digit (purp): Digitalis (purpurea)
Dulc: Dulcamara
***

E.
***

Elm: Bach Flower Remedy
Eupat: Eupatorium perfoliatum
***

F.
***

Ferr phos: Ferrum phosphoricum
Fluor ac: Fluoricum acidum
***

G.
***

Gels: Gelsemium
Gentian: Gentiana lutea
Germ: Germanium
Glon: Glonoine (Nitro-glycerine)
Gorse: Bach Flower Remedy
Graph: Graphites
***

H.
***

Ham: Hamamelis virginica
Heather: Bach Flower Remedy
Hell nig: Helleborus nigra
Hepar sulph: Hepar sulphuris calcareum
Holly: Bach Flower Remedy
Honeysuckle: Bach Flower Remedy
Hornbeam: Bach Flower Remedy
Hydro ac: Hydrocyanic acid
Hydro: Hydrophobinum
Hyos: Hyoscamus
Hyper: Hypericum
***

I.
***

Ign: Ignatia
Impatiens: Bach Flower Remedy
Iod: Iodum
Ipec: Ipecacuanha
Iris vers: Iris versicolor
***

K.
***

Kali bich: Kali bichromicum
Kali brom: Kali bromatum
Kali carb: Kali carbonicum
Kali iod: Kali iodatum
Kali phos: Kali phosphoricum
Kreos: Kreosotum
***

L.
***

Lach: Lachesis
Larch: Bach Flower Remedy
Ledum: Ledum
Lil tig: Lilium tigrinum
Lues: Lues (Syphilis)
Lyco: Lycopodium
Lyss: Lyssin(see Hydrophobinum)
***

M.
***

Mag carb: Magnesia carbonica
Mag mur: Magnesia muriaticum
Med: Medorrhinum
Meph puto: Mephitis puto (Skunk)
Melil: Melilotus
Merc sol: Mercurius solubilis
Merc viv: Mercurius vivus
Mimulus: Bach Flower Remedy
Mosch: Moschus
Mur ac: Muriaticum acidum
Mustard: Bach Flower Remedy
***

N.
***

Naja: Naja tripudians (cobra)
Nat mur: Natrum muriaticum
Nat sulph: Natrum sulphuricum
Nit ac: Nitricum acidum
Nux mosch: Nux moschata
Nux (vom): Nux vomica
***

O.
***

Oak: Bach Flower Remedy
Olive: Bach Flower Remedy
Onos: Onosmodium
Opium: Opium (poppy)
***

P.
***

Petro: Petroleum
Phos: Phosphorus
Phos ac: Phosphoricum acidum
Pine: Bach Flower Remedy
Plat: Platina (metal)
Plumb: Plumbum metallicum
Puls: Pulsatilla
Pyro: Pyrogenium
***

R.
***

Rad brom: Radium bromide
Rescue Remedy: Bach Flower Remedy
Rhodo: Rhododendron
Rhus tox: Rhus toxicodendron
Rockwater: Bach Flower Remedy
Ruta: Ruta graveolens
***

S.
***

Sabad: Sabadilla
Sali ac: Salicylic acid

Sang can: Sanguinaria canadensis
Scleranthus: Bach Flower Remedy
Sepia: Sepia
Sil: Silic(e)a (flint)
Spig: Spigelia
Staph: Staphysagria
Star of Bethlehem: Bach Flower Remedy
Stram: Stramonium
Strych: Strychninum
Sulph ac: Sulphuricum acidum
Sulph: Sulphur
***

T.
***

Tarent Hisp: Tarentula Hispania
Therid (cur): Theridion curassavicum (spider)
Thuja or Thuya: Thuja occidentalis (conifer)
Tub av: Tuberculinum aviaire
Tub (bov): Tuberculinum bovinum
***

V.
***

Ver alb: Veratrum album
Vervain: Bach Flower Remedy
Visc alb: Viscum album
***

W.
***

Walnut: Bach Flower Remedy
Water violet: Bach Flower Remedy
White Chestnut: Bach Flower Remedy

Wild oat: Bach Flower Remedy
Wild rose: Bach Flower Remedy
Willow: Bach Flower Remedy
***

Z.
***

Zinc: Zincum metallicum
Zinc sulph: Zinc sulphide
***

Bibliography.
***

http://en.wikipedia.org
www.abchomeopathy.com
www.cancernet.co.uk
www.clevelandclinicmeded.com
www.dermnet.com
www.druidry.org
www.emofree.com
www.elixiers.com
www.harvestfields.ca
www.healthy.net
www.helios.co.uk
www.herbs2000.com
www.holistc-home.com
www.homeoint.com
www.homeopath.moonfruit.com
www.homeopathyhome.com
www.hpathy.com
www.internethealthlibrary.com
www.mhra.gov.uk
www.lyghtforce.com
www.mediresource.sympatico.com
www.medicalhealthcures.com
www.ontariohomeopath.com
www.observer.guardian.co.uk
www.quantec.ch
www.realtime.net
www.ritecare.com
www.simillimum.com
www.spiritindia.com

www.wholehealthmd.com
***
Allport, R. Homeopathy for your Pets. Wigmore Publications Ltd, London. 2000.

Ball, P. The Essence of Tao. Arcturus Publishing, London. 2004.

Barnard, J. A Guide to the Bach Flower Remedies. C. W. Daniel, Saffron Walden. 2000.

Boericke, W. Homoeopathic Materia Medica. Homoeopathic Books Service, Kent. 1999.

Buber, M. I and Thou. Simon and Shuster, London. 1996.

Castro, M. The Complete Homeopathic Handbook. Pan Books Ltd, London. 1996.

Chapman, E. How to use the 12 Tissue Salts. Thorsons, UK. 1979.

Danciger, E. The Emergence of Homoeopathy. Century Hutchinson. London. 1987.

ECH General Assembly – XVII Symposium of GIRI 12-14 Nov 2004, Scientific Report.

Hahnemann and Dudgeon. Organon of Medicine. B. Jain Publishers, India. 1994.

Howard, J. Bach Flower Remedies for Women. C.W. Daniel Co. Ltd, Saffron Walden. 1992.

Hyne Jones, T.W. Dictionary of the Bach Flower Remedies. Saffron Walden, UK. 1995.

Juta, C.J.R.. Animal Homeopathy. BookSurge, USA. 2005.

Juta, C. J. Rupert. Better Sport with Homeopathy. Booksurge, USA. 2007.

Juta, C. J. Rupert. Can you Think, or are you Programmed?. Booksurge, USA. 2008.

Juta, C. J. Rupert. Modern Diseases and Disorders, and Homeopathy. Booksurge, USA. 2007.

Kent, J.T. Repertory of the Homeopathic Materia Medica. B. Jain Publishers Pty Ltd, New Delhi. 2004.

Lockie, A. The Family Guide to Homeopathy. Hamish Hamilton, London. 1998.

Macleod, G. Cats: Homeopathic Remedies. Mackays of Chatham, Kent. 1990.

Meyer, E. Family Encyclopaedia of Homeopathic Medicine. Bodywell Publishing. ?

Pert, J.C. Homeopathy. Wigmore Publications Ltd, London. 2002.

Morgan, F.E. Living the Martial Way. Barricade Books, New York. 1992.

Pacaud, D. Homeopathy Encyclopedia. Hachette, London. 2003.

Phatak, S.R. Materia Medica of Homeopathic Medicines. B.Jain Publishers, New Delhi. 2003.

Richardson-Boedler, C. Applying Homeopathy Bach Flower. B. Jain Publishers Ltd, New Delhi. 2004.

Williams, T. Complete Chinese Medicine. Element Books Ltd, Dorset. 1999.
***